ライフサイエンスのための英語

のための **英語**

English for Life Sciences
I. Essential Skills

I. 基本スキル編

萩原明子・小林 薫 編著

東京化学同人

序

2020 年は，新型コロナウイルスによる感染症（COVID-19）の全世界的な蔓延により，日常生活ばかりか私たちのもつ世界観まで大きく変わりました．世界が変われば，言語も変わります．2019 年までは，科学の世界以外では PCR という言葉を日常的に使用するということはありませんでしたが，現在では年齢層を問わず誰でも使用する日常語となりました．自然免疫，獲得免疫などの専門用語も頻繁に耳にするようになりました．ある意味で，生命科学が身近な存在になった年なのかもしれません．その一方で，情報技術の進んだこの時代でも，過去に伝染病が大流行したときと同じように，不正確な情報に振り回され，後世では不適切と判断されることが行われているかもしれないのも事実でしょう．

この教科書は，大学生が科学の知識を正確に得るために必要なスキルを習得するために企画されました．今は，理系の大学生だけでなく，他の分野の学生にとっても科学リテラシーが重要な時代です．科学分野の文献を正確に読み解く力は，これから起こりうるさまざまな問題に，個人あるいは社会のリーダーとして対処するためにも必要だと考えられます．科学の知識を得るために最も推奨される方法は，最新の論文を批判的な目で吟味しながら読むことです．それも，同じテーマで書かれた複数の論文を比較分析することが必要です．

大学生にとって論文を読むことはきわめて当たり前の行為です．しかし，現在出版されている論文のほとんどが英語で書かれており，日本語を母語とする大学生にとって難易度の高い行為になってしまっています．本来，科学論文は母語に関係なく読まれたり書かれたりするので，複雑な文構造や高度な言いまわしは必要ありません．基本的な英語の語彙と文法知識があれば読めるはずです．一方，科学的な素養は必要なので，英語の母語話者が英語で書かれているというだけの理由で科学論文をスラスラ読めるわけでもありません．たとえ母語が英語でなくても，科学英語は大学生がすでに身につけた基本的な英語力と科学の知識で十分に使いこなせるのです．

本書は，生命科学分野を学ぶ学生だけでなく，自然科学を専攻していない学生にとっても身近なトピックを扱い，知らず知らずのうちに英語で書かれた科学論文の読み方を身につけることを目標にしています．そのために，科学英語の読解スキルだけでなく，科学分野で使用される語彙の成り立ちや科学論文についての知識も多く含まれています．生命科学分野の語彙は綴りが複雑なだけでなく，発音も難しい場合があるため，音声を聞きながら学習することもできるように工夫しました．科学の情報を目からだけでなく耳から理解する習慣がつけば，将来，英語で学会発表をするときにも，テレビやインターネットで配信される科学ニュースを聞くときにも，海外の人々と日常の話題となっている環境問題や感染症などの話をするときにも，必ず役に立つことでしょう．

現代は世界の情報がリアルタイムで手に入る時代です．しかし，英語のスキルがないとその知識を直接得ることはできません．本書が正確な科学の情報を受取るためのスキルを習得する一助になることを執筆者一同，心から望んでいます．

2021 年 1 月

編者を代表して　萩　原　明　子

編　集

萩 原 明 子	東京薬科大学生命科学部 教授，Ph.D.（言語習得）
小 林 薫	東京農業大学生命科学部 教授，Ph.D.（応用言語学）

執　筆

小 林 薫	東京農業大学生命科学部 教授，Ph.D.（応用言語学）
権蛇 千香	マレーシア マラヤ大学大学院言語学研究科博士課程， 修士（生命科学）
内 藤 麻 緒	聖マリアンナ医科大学医学部 准教授，M.A.（言語教育）
萩 原 明 子	東京薬科大学生命科学部 教授，Ph.D.（言語習得）
星 野 裕 子	前 東京薬科大学生命科学部 教授，M.A.（言語教育）
Andrea D. Little	東京薬科大学生命科学部 非常勤講師，M.Sc.（科学英語教育）

（五十音順）

ナレーター（音声データ）

Andrea D. Little	東京薬科大学生命科学部 非常勤講師，M.Sc.（科学英語教育）
Eden M. Foster	米国 ウィスコンシン大学マディソン校
Joel Y. Foster	米国 ウィスコンシン大学マディソン校
Naomi K. Foster	米国 ウィスコンシン大学マディソン校

科 学 監 修

井 上 英 史	東京薬科大学名誉教授，薬学博士

本書の使い方

本書の目的

　本書は医学，薬学，生物学，農学などの生命科学分野を専攻する学生を対象とし，大学教養分野の英語と専門分野で使用する英語の橋渡しをするものです．本書には三つの目的があります．第一に科学英語における機能表現の習得，第二にスタディースキル（読解スキルと語彙学習ストラテジー）の紹介と実践，第三に生命科学で使用する多くの語彙に含まれる接頭辞・接尾辞・語根の習得です．

1．科学英語における機能表現の習得

　学生の皆さんが研究室に配属された後に読み書きする論文には，目的に応じて使われる決まり文句や文型などの機能表現が多く見られます．たとえば［用語の定義をする］，［結果を比較する］，［例示する］，［方法，手順を表す］などの目的のために使用される表現は，分野を問わず文献の中でもよく使われます．本書では，これらの機能表現を，生命科学分野のテキストや語彙を使って提示し，さまざまな練習問題を通してそれらの使用法（パラフレーズを含む）を習得することを目指します．

2．スタディースキル

　本書では，以下の二つのスタディースキルを身につけることを目標としています．

　a．読解スキル（リーディング＋ノートテイキング）　効率のよいリーディングとは，文字情報を目で追うだけではありません．発音と組合わせ，テキストの構成を理解して初めて内容理解が可能です．さらに読んだ内容を記憶にとどめ後日の復習に備えるためにはノートを取る（ノートテイキング）のが効果的です．本書では，まずはキーワードを聞き取り，書き取るこ

とから始め，構成理解，内容理解を経てテキストのそれぞれの段落の主旨（main idea），全体を通しての論旨（thesis）を読み取り，最終的にノートテイキングをします．

　b．語彙学習ストラテジー　言語の基本は単語です．多くの語を知れば知るほどその言語を流ちょうに操ることができます．本書では，語彙学習ストラテジーを身につけるために有効な学習法を紹介します．

3．生命科学分野の接頭辞・接尾辞・語根の習得

　私たちは初めて見る漢字に遭遇したとき，まず部首を見て，［ニクヅキ］であれば身体が関係しているかな，とか［リッシンベン］であれば感情に関わる意味かな，と想像します．漢字の部首に相当するものを英語では語の形態素（接頭辞・接尾辞・語根）といいます．特に生命科学分野ではギリシャ語やラテン語の接頭辞，接尾辞，語根から成り立っている語が多く存在し，それらの構成素から意味を予測することが可能です．本書では，特に生命科学分野の語に多く見られる接頭辞，接尾辞，語根などを学習することによって，生命科学関連の語彙を増やすことを目指します．

本書の構成

　本書は Study Guide，Textbook（六つの Unit），Workbook（六つの Unit）から成り立っています．

Study Guide	各 Unit の構成
Textbook	**I．Reading and listening**
	1 Pre-reading activities
	2 Reading text
	3 Understanding the structure
	4 Reading for details
	5 Note-taking
	II．Language focus
	6 Sentence patterns
	7 Application
	III．Vocabulary and vocabulary learning skills
	8 Words in the reading text
	9 Word-formation
	IV．Scientific communication
	10 Basics
	11 Exercise
Workbook	**1** Reading
	2 Language focus
	3 Vocabulary
	4 Reading glossary
	5 Word-formation samples

ノートを取ることの利点
1. 必要な情報を整理することができる
2. 内容に集中することによって理解が深まる
3. 学習した内容が頭に残る

論文を正確に理解するにはノートを取って情報を整理することが重要です．

Study Guide

Study Guide では各 Unit に繰返し出てくる概念と具体的な学習法を説明しています．たとえば topic sentence, main idea や thesis という用語は，多くの Unit で出てきますが，Unit の中では説明していません．Study Guide では，これらの概念と，ノートテイキングの方法，語彙学習法，文型を利用したパラフレーズの方法など学習法について説明しています．

Textbook

六つの Unit からなり，各 Unit は **1**〜**11** の要素からなっています．

I. Reading and listening

リーディングは目だけで行うものと思っていませんか．実は，リーディングを行う際，頭の中では文字情報を音韻情報に変えています．黙読しているつもりでぶつぶつと音読をしていることがあるでしょう．その際，単語をすらすら発音したり，一つの文章を正しく区切ったりできなければ読むスピードが遅くなったり，文意を正しく読み取れなくなったりします．本書では，速いスピードで正しく読む（流ちょうに読む）ことを目指して，リーディングはリスニングから入ります．続いてテキストの構成と内容理解，次のセクションで学習する機能表現にふれ，最後にテキストの内容をノートテイキングによってまとめます．以下の手順で学習しましょう．

1 Pre-reading activities

Discussion と Listening activities があります．Discussion をすることにより，どんな内容のテキストを読むのか，頭の中でストーリーをつくってみましょう．続く Listening activities ではすべてを聞き取ろうとせず，まず keyword を聞き取ってみましょう．その後，本文のページに行き，音声を模して音読してみましょう．教科書を見ないで行うシャドーイングも効果的です．

2 Reading text

リーディングの本文です．

3 Understanding the structure

本格的な読みに入る前に，まず本文を一読し構成を把握しましょう．再度本文を読み，keyword を読み取りましょう．それぞれの keyword がどの段落（paragraph）に出てきたかも確認しておきましょう．Listening activities で聞き取った keyword と比較してみましょう．

4 Reading for details

このセクションでは各 Unit の機能表現を学習します．内容について理解を深め，応用問題にも挑戦します．

5 Note-taking

Unit ごとに，本文のそれぞれの段落の主旨（main idea），本文全体の論旨（thesis）を確認します．

II. Language focus

Language focus では生命科学分野の文献の中で使用される機能表現を学習します（ものの定義のしかた，分類表現，計測の表現など）．基本的な学習の手順は以下のとおりです．

6 Sentence patterns

科学英語で頻繁に使用される機能表現を学び，その意味と目的を確認します．まず，四角で囲んである部分の解説を読み内容を理解してください．ここで紹介されている sentence patterns はその Unit のテーマとなる機能表現の基本形なので覚えましょう．

7 Application

ここでは Sentence patterns で学んだ文型を使用して，文をつくったり，文を完成させたりする練習問題を通して，英作文の力を養います．書くだけではなく音声を聞いて問いに答える問題もあります．それぞれの Unit で紹介されている機能表現を読んだり，書いたりするだけでなく，会話の中でも使ってみてください．より専門的な例文を使って，文の構造を確認したり，パラフレーズをしたりする練習もあります．

〈文型ノート〉〈文法ノート〉 その機能表現を使用する際に知っておくと便利な知識は，囲み記事の〈文型ノート〉〈文法ノート〉にあります．この教科書でふれていなくても，授業で科学英語についての知識を学んだら，まとめておく習慣をつけましょう．

III. Vocabulary and vocabulary learning skills

8 Words in the reading text

このセクションでは本文に出てきた生命科学の各分野でよく使われる語彙を学習します．単語の品詞を確認したり，語彙の定義を書いたりしながら，語彙を増やす努力をしましょう．文章をすらすら読むためには，文の主語と動詞を素早く正確に読み取ることが必要です．長い文の場合，一見してどこまでが主語か，どれが動詞かがわかりにくいことがあります．文の構造がスムーズにわかるようになるまで，意識的に品詞や意味を考えながら，語彙を学びましょう．

9 Word-formation

自然科学の研究発表には英語が使われます．論文も英語で書かれ，国際学会での発表も英語で行われます．ところが日本の大学では，一部の大学を除くと専門分野を学ぶときに英語ではなく日本語を使用しています．世界の多くの国の学生が母語ではなく英語で専門分野を学んでいることを考えると，日本で科学を学ぶ学生は真剣に英語の科学語彙を学ぶ必要があります．

はじめに，科学語彙の〈語の成り立ち〉を学んで，新しい語が出てきたときに正確に意味を類推するための方法を紹介します．この方法は，語の形態素，その中でも，特に接辞（affix）を体系的に学び，複雑に見える専門用語を学ぶ方法です．日本人が漢字の部首の意味や漢字の組合わせから，語の意味を類推することと似ています．特に接辞の中でも接頭辞（prefix），接尾辞（suffix）について紹介しています．それぞれの接辞を使った語の例を表に示しています．接辞がどのように語を形成するか，その接辞の意味と使われ方を覚えましょう．接辞を用いた練習問題もあります．長い語もパーツにわけて意味を考えれば，意味が正確にわかるだけでなく，記憶することにもつながります．

IV. Scientific communication

10 Basics

皆さんはもう研究室に所属していますか．たとえ先輩からひき継いだものでも，自分自身のテーマで研究を始めたら，皆さんはもう立派な研究者です．苦労や失敗を重ねた末にまとめた自分の研究を，学会に出席して発表し，それについて他の研究者からアドバイスをもらったり，ときには議論をしたりと，研究者同士のコミュニケーションの輪の中に身をおくことになり

ます．生命科学分野は，まさに日進月歩の，世界的に注目されている分野です．研究者同士，知見を共有し切磋琢磨する際の共通語は英語です．このセクションでは全 Unit を通して科学コミュニケーションに加わるための基礎知識を紹介します．

11 Exercise

10 で得られた知識を確認するために練習問題を解いてみましょう．

Workbook

Textbook で学習したことを強化するための各 Unit ごとの練習問題と，各 Unit のおもな単語のリストから成っています．練習問題は授業の復習に，単語リストはテキストの文脈の中での単語の意味の確認に使用してください．

1 Reading

内容理解を深める問題です．リスニングの記述問題もあります．4 技能のスキル向上につながるように工夫した問題が揃っています．

2 Language focus

機能表現の応用問題です．機能表現の聞き取りを強化するためのリスニング問題もあります．実際に科学論文で使用された文を使った練習問題も含まれます．

3 Vocabulary

Reading で学習した語彙の機能表現，語形成（word-formation）の応用問題のほかリスニングの書き取り問題があります．

4 Reading glossary

Textbook の本文に使用されている語彙のリストです．意味を考えながら音声を聞き，自分で発音しながら学習しましょう．

5 Word-formation samples

Textbook の Word-formation の表の中で例として紹介されている語彙のリストです．日本語での意味を確認しましょう．科学語彙は，日本語のカタカナ読みとは発音が大きく異なるので，アクセントの位置に気をつけながら発音の練習もしましょう．

◀)) 音声データについて

本書付属の“音声データ”を本書購入者本人に限り，下記の要領で取得できます．

1. 音声データの内容

　録音内容：Textbook 各 Unit の Reading，7B，7C
　　　　　　Workbook　各 Unit の 4. Reading glossary，5. Word-formation samples
　ナレーター：Andrea D. Little，Eden M. Foster，Joel Y. Foster，Naomi K. Foster
　ファイル形式：MP3

2. 音声の再生の仕方

　スマートフォンで QR コードを読み取る方法と，パソコンで全音声データを一括ダウンロードする方法があります．

2・1　QR コードを読み取る（インターネットに接続した状態で）

　お手持ちのスマートフォンで右のような QR コードを読み取っていただけましたら，直ちに対応箇所の再生が始まります．

◀)) Track 0

2・2　音声データを一括ダウンロードする

　MP3 形式の音声ファイルを ZIP 形式で提供いたします．すべての音声データを一括ダウンロードすることができます．下記の手順，動作環境でダウンロードし，パソコンで再生してご利用ください．録音時間　約 100 分

　[ダウンロードの手順]
　1）パソコンで東京化学同人のホームページにアクセスし，書名検索などにより，“ライフサイエンスのための英語 I. 基本スキル編”の画面を表示させる．
　2）画面最後尾の ［音声ダウンロード］ をクリックし，下記のユーザー名およびパスワードを入力する．（本書購入者本人以外は使用できません．図書館での利用は館内での使用に限ります．）

　　　　　　　　　　ユーザー名：**JFA5Efr4**
　　　　　　　　　　パスワード：**s7mPWu5B**

　[サインイン] を選択すると，ダウンロードが始まる．

　※　ファイルは ZIP 形式で圧縮されていますので，解凍ソフトで解凍のうえ，ご利用ください．

[動作環境]

　音声データのダウンロードおよび再生には，下記の動作環境を推奨します．この動作環境を満たしていないパソコンでは正常にダウンロードおよび再生ができない場合がありますので，ご了承ください．

OS：　Microsoft Windows 10，Mac OS X，11（日本語版サービスパックなどは最新版）
推奨ブラウザ：　Microsoft Edge，Microsoft Internet Explorer，Safari など
コンテンツ再生：　Microsoft Windows Media Player，Quick Time Player など

3. 講義で使用する（CD プレイヤーで再生する）場合

　CD プレイヤーなどで再生する場合には，パソコン上で適切なアプリケーション（Windows Media Player など）を用いて，オーディオ CD（データ CD ではない）を作成していただく必要があります．CD は 1 枚では入りきらないので 2 枚ご準備ください．オーディオ CD の作成の仕方は，各アプリケーションの説明書でご確認ください．弊社でのお客様ごとの個別対応はいたしかねますのでご了承ください．

教員用資料

　本書採用の教員に限り，以下のものを東京化学同人より入手できます（東京化学同人 営業部にご連絡ください．info@tkd-pbl.com）

① Textbook の解答・解説
② Workbook の問題の音声と解答

目　　次

Study Guide

科学英語習得のための効果的な学習法の手引き

この教科書では，科学英語を通してさまざまな学習スキルを身につけることを目標としています．この Study Guide では，繰返し出てくる概念を A. Reading strategies，B. Vocabulary learning strategies に大別し，説明します．次に C. Paraphrasing では，科学論文を実際に読み，その内容をレポートにまとめたり引用したりする際に欠かせないパラフレーズする（別の表現で言い換える）スキルを説明します．論文の剽窃がよく話題に上りますが，パラフレーズは不適切な引用をさけるためには重要なスキルです．

A. Reading strategies

文章の構成：Thesis statement, topic sentence と main idea

アカデミックな文章はたいていの場合，introduction，body，conclusion の三部構成になっています．Introduction には著者がその文章で伝えたいこと（thesis）を要約した文があり，それを thesis statement とよびます．下の introduction paragraph を読んで thesis statement を確認しましょう．

DNA is often called the blueprint of life. Reading the sequence of DNA allows you to see the characteristics of an animal. If you analyze DNA, it is possible to diagnose diseases. In the 1980s, a technique called PCR method which makes multiple copies of a specific DNA segment in a test tube was developed. Since then, PCR has been used in many areas of biology and medicine to study characteristics of organisms. Interestingly enough, it is not only the field of life sciences where PCR is used, but also the field of history where it is used to solve mysteries of the past. 〈Unit 2 Reading より〉

下線部が thesis statement で thesis は "PCR is used not only in the field of life sciences but also in the field of history." です．

Conclusion では文章全体の内容を振返ります．たいていの場合，確認のために thesis statement が再び出てきます．Unit 2 の最後の段落のどこに thesis statement が出てくるか探してみましょう．

Body は複数の段落（paragraph）で構成され，それぞれの paragraph は一つのまとまった考え（main idea）を伝えます．Main idea は，しばしば topic sentence とよばれる文によって表されます．Topic sentence は多くの場合，paragraph の最初か最後に置かれます．下の paragraph で確認しましょう．

PCR was also used to investigate Ötzi, the iceman who was found in the Tirolean Alps in 1991. Ötzi is a natural mummy that was well preserved in a glacier for a long time. Carbon dating revealed that he died more than 5000 years ago. His possessions indicate that he was a wealthy man. CT scans and X-rays showed that he had been killed with an arrow. However, who he was genetically or if he is linked to any modern humans remained a mystery. To unravel this, scientists used PCR and found that he is an ancestor of modern Europeans who live in Austria. The genetic investigation even identified 19 living people who are related to Ötzi. 〈Unit 2 Reading より〉

下線部が topic sentence で main idea は "PCR was also used to investigate Ötzi, an iceman." です．

Outline（アウトライン）

　テキスト中の情報をノートに整理すると理解が深まります．整理する方法の一つとして outline 作成があります．paragraph の main idea とそれを裏付ける supporting details（数字で示している項目）を拾っていくと outline が仕上がります．上の introduction の paragraph の outline は次のようになります．

PCR is used to identify an organism not only in the field of life sciences but also in the field of history.

　　1．PCR is a method to make multiple copies of a DNA segment.

　　2．With PCR, researchers can study characteristics of organisms.

　　3．PCR is now used in many fields including biology, medicine and history.

Note-taking（ノートテイキング・ノートを取る）

　Outline はノートの形にまとめると（ノートテイキング）効率的です．情報を整理し，キーポイントを自分の言葉でまとめます．

1．まず紙に右のような枠を作ります．
　　　　　　　　　　　　（ステップ 1）

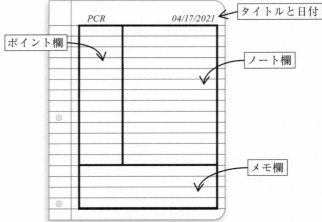

2．テキストを読みながらノート欄にノートを取っていきます（ステップ 2）．

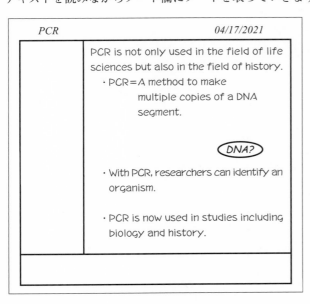

　　1．Paragraph の main idea を書く．

　　2．Main idea の根拠を箇条書きで書く．

　　3．Outline も可．

　　4．図やイラスト，グラフも可．

　　5．自分が理解できなかったこともメモする → 教員・友達に確認．

　　6．予習の段階からノートを作成し，授業中，授業後にも書き入れる．

　　7．省略記号の使用も可．

　　8．項目ごとに余白をつくる → 後でノートの追加ができる．

3. ポイント欄にはキーワードや重要ポイントを書込みます（ステップ3）. ポイント欄は, 後日, 復習の際に使用することができます.

```
 PCR                              04/17/2021

 What is      PCR is not only used in the field of life
 PCR?         sciences but also in the field of history.
                     · PCR=A method to make
                        multiple copies of a DNA
                        segment.
                                      (DNA?)
 What can
 you do       · With PCR, researchers can identify an
 with PCR?    organism.

 In what
 fields is    · PCR is now used in studies including
 PCR          biology and history.
 used?

```

• ポイント欄にキーワード・キーフレーズを書く.

• 復習に使えるように, "What is PCR?" などと疑問文にするのもよい.

4. 最後に一番下の枠内に疑問点, 自分の感想, 学んだことなどを自由にメモします（ステップ4）.

```
 PCR                              04/17/2021

 What is      PCR is not only used in the field of life
 PCR?         sciences but also in the field of history.
                     · PCR=A method to make
                        multiple copies of a DNA
                        segment.
                                      (DNA?)
 What can
 you do       · With PCR, researchers can identify an
 with PCR?    organism.

 In what
 fields is    · PCR is now used in studies including
 PCR used?    biology and history.

 PCR makes multiple copies of a DNA segment and makes
 it easy for researchers to study it. PCR is used to identify
 an organism not only in the field of life sciences but in the
 field of history.

 DNA: deoxyribonucleic acid  デオキシリボ核酸  染色体
 の重要部分で遺伝子の本体となる
```

• メモ欄にはメモや thesis, 自分が学んだことなどを自由にメモする.

5. 出来上がったこのノートは後日，折りたたんでポイント欄を
   見ながら復習に使うことができます．

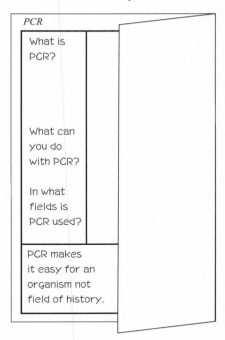

6. ノートを取る際，省略記号を使うと便利です．下の表は英語でよく使用される省略記号です．専門用語
   の中には略語が存在するものもあります（例：表中 17-19）．どんどん取り入れましょう．

1	with	w/		11	A から B になる，A の結果 B になる	A ⟶ B
2	without	w/o				
3	because	b/c		12	A の原因は B である	A ⟵ B
4	important	imp.		13	より多い	>
5	for example	e.g.,		14	より少ない	<
6	つまり　that is	i.e.,		15	よって・だから・結果として	∴
7	最高で	max		16	理由は〜	∵
8	最低で	min		17	red blood cell	RBC
9	million	mil.		18	white blood cell	WBC
10	billion	bil.		19	immunoglobulin	Ig

B. Vocabulary learning strategies

　　単語を学習するときどんな工夫をしていますか．一般的に，単語学習ストラテジーには脳内の処理が浅
いものと深いものの二種類あります．脳内処理が浅いものは，［見る］，［書く］，［発音する］など工夫があ

まり必要ないもの，脳内処理が深いものは［イメージを描く（イメージストラテジー）］［連想する（連想ストラテジー）］［作文する（作文ストラテジー）］［接頭辞・接尾辞に分ける（語形成ストラテジー）］など頭を使う必要があるもので，単語を長期記憶に保存するには脳内処理が深いものが有効とされています．ここではイメージストラテジー，連想ストラテジー，作文ストラテジーの紹介をします．語形成ストラテジーは，医学・生物学系の単語には特に役立つストラテジーなので，本書の各ユニットで紹介しています．

Image strategy（イメージストラテジー）

　学習する単語（目標単語）を単語の意味を表すイメージ（写真，絵，図，心象）と結びつけるのが効果的だということは多くの研究者によって実証されています．このストラテジーは，特に理系の英単語を学習するときに役立ちます．なぜなら理系，特に生物系の英単語は生物の部位を表すもの，何かの現象や，生物学的・化学的なプロセスを示すものが多いからです．イメージといっても具体的なものから心象的なものまでさまざまです．以下，おもなものを五つ紹介します．

1. 図絵：単語の示す意味の具体的なイメージ，または抽象的なものについては自分の頭の中にあるイメージ．

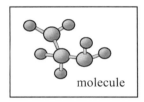

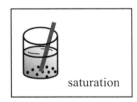

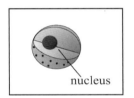

2. 個人的経験：語の示す意味について自分の個人的経験と結びつけてイメージを描く．

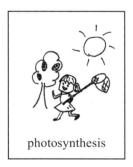

例：'photosynthesis'（光合成）と，子どものころに森に虫取りに行ったとき，木の葉を見て光合成について考えた思い出のイメージを結びつける．

3. スペリングのイメージ：スペリングの形がもつイメージと語の意味を結びつける．

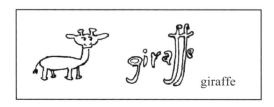

4. 語呂合わせ: 語の発音と似ている日本語の語（意味的に関連があるとなおよい）の音と意味をイメージしながら学習する.

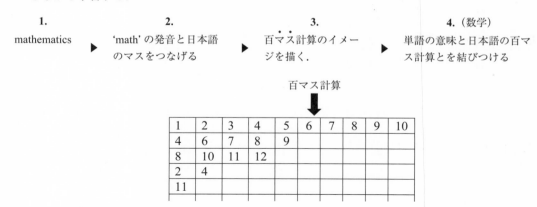

1.		2.		3.		4.（数学）
mathematics	▶	'math' の発音と日本語のマスをつなげる	▶	百マス計算のイメージを描く.	▶	単語の意味と日本語の百マス計算とを結びつける

百マス計算

1	2	3	4	5	6	7	8	9	10
4	6	7	8	9					
8	10	11	12						
2	4								
11									

5. 良いイメージ・悪いイメージ: 語の意味が良いイメージか悪いイメージかを考えるのも役立ちます.

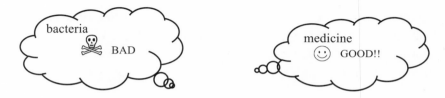

bacteria ☠ BAD

medicine ☺ GOOD!!

Association strategy（連想ストラテジー）

　学びたい語の意味から他の語を連想し, 語のネットワークをつくります. 図（a）は pathogen（病原体）という語を中心とした意味のネットワーク, 図（b）は female（女性）の同義語と対義語のネットワーク, 図（c）は funnel（じょうご）と同じ実験器具のカテゴリーに属す語, つまり包摂関係のネットワークを連想したものです. これらのネットワークの大小は問いませんが, 英語であること, 自分で考えることが大事です（考える過程が記憶につながります）.

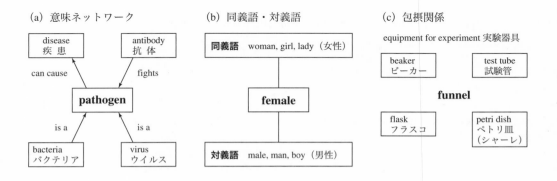

(a) 意味ネットワーク

| disease 疾患 | | antibody 抗体 |
| can cause | | fights |
| **pathogen** |
| is a | | is a |
| bacteria バクテリア | | virus ウイルス |

(b) 同義語・対義語

| 同義語 | woman, girl, lady （女性） |
| **female** |
| 対義語 | male, man, boy （男性） |

(c) 包摂関係

equipment for experiment 実験器具

| beaker ビーカー | test tube 試験管 |
| flask フラスコ | petri dish ペトリ皿 （シャーレ） |

funnel

Composition strategy（作文ストラテジー）

　学びたい語を使って作文をするとその語の意味や用法を深く考えることにつながります. たとえば, pesticide, atmosphere, obesity, longevity を学びたいときは, それぞれを使って自分で英文を作成します.

Many farmers use **pesticides** to increase the yield of crops.
Earth's **atmosphere** contains nitrogen, oxygen, argon, and carbon dioxide.
Obesity can be a cause of many deadly diseases.
The family is famous for their **longevity**.

学びたい語を複数使用して一つの英文をつくることも脳内の深い処理になります.

Pesticides in the **atmosphere** can cause air pollution.

自分で作文した場合,適切な文かどうかが気になります.インターネットや辞書などで確認しましょう.

Word formation strategy（語形成ストラテジー）

　語の接頭辞,接尾辞と語根を知ると,知らない語でも意味がある程度予測できます.これは漢字の部首を知っていると知らない漢字の意味がある程度予測できるのと同じことです.特に生命科学関連の専門用語は,接頭辞＝prefix,接尾辞＝suffix（これらを合わせて接辞＝affix）,語根（root）に分けられるものが多いので,それらを学習することは語彙を増やすうえで有効です.下の例を見てみましょう.

transplantation
trans（across 向こう側へ）＋ plantation（the noun form of 'to plant 植える'）── 移植

chlorophyll
chloro（green 緑）＋ phyll（leaf 葉）　葉緑素

辞書を見ると以下のような情報が載っています.L はラテン語の affix, G はギリシャ語の affix です.語彙学習ストラテジーとしては,どの接辞が L か G か区別して覚える必要はありませんが,辞書に出てくる情報として記憶にとどめておくと便利です.

organism ── organ（L. or G. tool 道具）＋ suffix -ism（suffix to form a noun）
　働くもののあつまり＝生命体

defend ── de-（L. off 遠ざける）＋ fend（L. to strike 攻撃する）
　撃退する

recognition ── re-（L. again 再び）＋ cogn（L. to know 知る）＋ -tion（suffix to form a noun）
　再び知ること＝認識する

disinfectant ── dis-（L. taking apart バラバラにする）＋ infect（L. to infect 感染する）＋
　　　　　　　　　　　　　　　　　　　　　　　　　　　　　　-ant（suffix to form a noun）
　感染を分解する＝殺菌/消毒

macrophage ── macro-（G. large 大きい）＋ phage（G. to eat 食べる）
　たくさん食べる＝マクロファージ

C. Paraphrasing （パラフレーズ・別の表現で言い換えること）

　論文を読む目的は研究課題に関しての知識を広めることですが，読んだ論文から得た情報を自分の論文に引用することがあります．科学研究は，これまでの研究を通して蓄積された知見に基づいてのみ新しい発見が可能であり，ほかの研究者の書いた論文を引用するのは，論文を書くうえで最も基本的なことといえます．他の研究者の業績を引用するときには，正しい方法で引用しなければ，剽窃という研究不正に問われる危険性があります．ここでは，論文の引用方法の種類，引用する際に注意すべきこと，正しく引用するために必須のパラフレーズの方法について簡単に説明します．

　まず引用の方法は，大きく二通りあります．

　一つは，著者の言葉遣いをそのまま引用する［直接引用］という方法です．この形で引用する場合は，引用する箇所を引用符（quotation marks）で囲み，引用する文献のページ（出典）を入れて，どこから引用したか，具体的に示します．文学作品を批評するときにはこの方法が必須なため，文学の論文では，引用符で囲む比較的短い引用だけでなく，block quote という塊で引用する方法さえあります．

　二つ目の方法は，自分の言葉で引用元の内容を完全にパラフレーズし，出典情報を入れた［間接引用］というものです．科学論文では，引用のほとんどは［間接引用］によるもので，パラフレーズするために元の文章を完全に別の言葉に言い換えたり，一つの論文の内容を一言（one phrase）で要約（summarize）したりする場合がほとんどです．

　元の文を十分にパラフレーズしないで引用すると，［剽窃/盗用（plagiarism）］とされることがあります．過去には，研究不正の一つとして剽窃を問われ学位を剥奪された研究者が何人もいます．現在は，インターネットが学術情報をつないでおり，以前よりも剽窃のチェックが容易にできるようになっています．学生の中には，軽い気持ちでインターネット上にある情報をレポートにそのままコピーして，引用情報をつけずに，あるいは，不正確に引用しそれを自分のレポートとして提出する人がいるかもしれませんが，それらはすべて剽窃であり，研究不正になります．英語論文の場合，英語の知識が十分でないために不適切な引用をし，それを指摘されることがあるかもしれません．これらを避けるためには，間接引用に必須のスキルである，パラフレーズの方法を学ぶことが重要です．

　パラフレーズにはいろいろな方法があります．使用されている単語を別のものに変えたり，文型を変えたりしてほぼ同じ内容が示せるようにする，などです．語彙，文型を変えて文を書き直すには，少し勉強が必要なので，この教科書では，Language focus のセクションで，さまざまな意味を表す機能表現を学習します．一つの文型で書かれた文を別の文型で書き直す練習を重ねれば，研究室で論文の内容を発表するときに，論文の丸写しを避けることができることはもとより，将来自分が論文を書くときにも使える作文の技能につながります．

> **よく使われるパラフレーズの方法**
> 1. 元の文と違った語彙を使用する
> 2. 元の文と違った文型を使用する
> 3. 語彙も文型も違うものにする

この教科書の練習問題では，おもに［違った文型を使用する］ことによってパラフレーズを練習します．実際に論文を引用するときには，単なるパラフレーズだけでは十分ではなく，内容を要約するスキルも必要ですが，要約するときにも，文型の練習は役立ちます．

パラフレーズの例：

元の文：

"Limonin is a phytonutrient found in most citrus fruits. Natural sources of limonin include oranges, grapefruits, lemons, and limes." （www.limonin.com から引用）

1. 単語を変える：

   Limonin <u>refers to</u> a phytonutrient <u>contained</u> in most citrus fruits.

2. 二つの文を繋げる：

   Limonin <u>refers to</u> a phytonutrient <u>that can be found</u> in citrus fruits such as oranges and lemons.

3. 文の構造を完全に変える：

   Many citrus fruits such as grapefruits, oranges, limes and lemons contain a phytonutrient called Limonin.

文の書き換えを苦手にしている学生が多いようですが，ちょっとした工夫で比較的容易にできるようになります．将来，剽窃の疑いをかけられないためにも，今から練習に励みましょう．

Textbook

聴解，読解，文型，語彙の学習と練習問題

Unit 1
Defining
What is science ?　　Science is ⋯

Unit 1 では以下の事柄を学びます.

Ⅰ．Reading and listening

Topic 1　Limburger Cheese and Mosquitoes
　　　　　"臭いチーズと蚊"

1 Pre-reading activities

2 Reading text

3 Understanding the structure

4 Reading for details：Understanding definitions
物や事柄の定義を理解する

5 Note-taking：Finding the main ideas in a text
文章中からメインアイディア（主旨）を見つける

Ⅱ．Language focus

6 Sentence patterns：Defining matter or a concept
物や事柄を定義する

7 Application：Using the sentence patterns

Ⅲ．Vocabulary and vocabulary learning skills

8 Words in the reading text

9 Word-formation：Prefixes related to numbers
語形成：数に関連する接頭辞を学ぶ

Ⅳ．Scientific communication

10 Academic organizations
研究に関わる情報の伝達と共有の方法を知る

11 Exercise

Workbook（Unit 1）▶ p. W 3

I   Reading and listening

Topic 1   **Limburger Cheese and Mosquitoes**

1   Pre-reading activities

1 A   Discuss the following with your partner.

1. Have you ever seen mosquitoes land on a piece of cheese?

2. What do you think attracts mosquitoes to humans?

3. Mosquitoes kill millions of people every year. Is this statement true or false?

1 B   Listening activities   (Track 1)

1. Listen to the recording and write the keywords from the text.

2. Listen again, paying attention to intonation, pronunciation, and pauses.

3. Read the text below aloud with the recording.

2   Reading text   (Track 1)

◀)) Track 1

Topic 1

Limburger Cheese and Mosquitoes[1), 2)]

When I think of summer, I think of fireworks and camping, but I also think of itchy mosquito bites and their annoying buzzing as I try to sleep. Mosquitoes aren't just annoying, however; they are responsible for transmitting some of the deadliest diseases around the world and killing millions of people each year. The diseases include malaria, dengue fever, Japanese encephalitis, and the West Nile Virus. Have you ever wondered what attracts mosquitoes to humans or why some people seem to get bitten more often than others?

Mosquitoes are hematophagous insects. Hematophagous means subsisting on blood, so mosquitoes are insects that feed on blood. To find potential blood hosts, mosquitoes rely on both their vision and their sense of smell. And, of course, there are a variety of factors that make some human hosts stand out more than others. For example, mosquitoes can see us more easily if we are wearing noticeable colors such as red, navy blue, or black. Certain odors, too, including those of the carbon dioxide we exhale and our chemical-laden sweat, enable mosquitoes to track us down. Bigger people and pregnant women who exhale larger volumes of CO_2, as well as people who are exercising vigorously and building up heat and lactic acid, are easier to find and are more likely to be bitten. Mosquitoes are also attracted to odors associated with certain body regions and types of skin bacteria. For instance, the distinctive odor of *Brevibacterium epidermidis*, which is a coryneform bacteria that lives between our toes and causes foot odor, is especially appealing to the insect.

Given how deadly mosquito-borne diseases are, wouldn't it be great if we could harness our smelly foot odor to make a mosquito trap? This is not really a far-fetched notion. Researchers are attempting to develop odor-baited traps that can control mosquitoes and reduce the transmission of malaria. Interestingly, one odor that has been used is Limburger cheese.

Why cheese? Scientists have found that Limburger, a pungent cheese with an odor remarkably like smelly feet, can be used to attract *Anopheles gambiae*, the chief malaria vector in Africa. (A vector is an organism that transmits a disease.) This isn't really surprising because *Brevibacterium linens*, a microorganism from the same genus as *B. epidermidis*, is used to make the cheese and is responsible for its smell. Limburger cheese ripens in a warm, moist environment, which is much like that of the environment between our toes where the bacteria *B. epidermidis* thrive. Scientists hypothesize that the similar odors of Limburger cheese and our feet are due to the comparable environments. In addition, gas chromatographic analyses have confirmed that the carboxylic fatty acid compositions of the odor of the cheese and toe-nail scrapings are very similar. A group of researchers, in fact, found one species of mosquito, *A. gambiae* sensu stricto, is attracted to synthetic blends of those acids.

Drawing on this evidence, researchers in Africa have been experimenting with odor-baited traps as potential tools for monitoring mosquito vectors of malaria and similarly transmitted diseases. One researcher in Kenya developed a simple trap using Limburger cheese, heat, and moisture that successfully attracted mosquitoes. This raises the possibility that similar, inexpensive traps could be used in the future to trap mosquitoes both in homes and on a larger scale.

* sensu stricto (Latin) = in a strict sense

3 Understanding the structure

3 A Text analysis

1. How many paragraphs are there? There are （   ) paragraphs.

2. Read the text once again and write the keywords from the text. Compare with the answers in "1 B Listening activities."

> [ ]

3. Choose one keyword from the above list and discuss it with your partner.

Your partner： What word did you choose?

You： I chose （   ).

Your partner： Can you explain the word?

You：＿＿＿＿＿＿＿＿＿＿＿＿＿＿＿＿＿＿＿＿＿＿＿＿

3 B Skimming

1. What is the purpose of this text?

> [ ]

2. What did the scientists find?

> [ ]

4 Reading for details： Understanding definitions

4 A Words in context

1. Find and circle the following terms in the text.

2. Write the description for each term in the boxes below.

mosquito

> [ ]

malaria

> [ ]

Anopheles gambiae

```



```

vector

```



```

Limburger cheese

```



```

Brevibacterium epidermidis

```



```

4 B Scanning： Where can you find the answers to the questions below？ Underline the parts in the text. Discuss the answers with your partner.

1. What makes some people more attractive to mosquitoes than other people？

2. Why do mosquitoes come close to Limburger cheese？

3. Describe the mosquito trap being developed by researchers.

4 C Schematization and extension： Work in groups. Discuss the answers to the following questions.

1. What might the mosquito trap look like？ Draw an image of the mosquito trap described in the reading.

```




```

2. What do *Brevibacterium epidermidis* and *Brevibacterium linens* have in common？

5 Note-taking：Finding the main ideas in a text

5 A Read the **Study Guide**（p. 2）and learn about the following terms. Write a definition for each in English.

1. Topic sentence_____

2. Main idea_____

3. Thesis_____

5 B Read each paragraph carefully and underline the part which contains its main idea.

文型ノート：定義

　論文や論文要旨（abstract）の背景を説明する部分によく使用される英語表現に［定義］があります．定義には最低でも三つの要素（［定義する語］［定義するものを含む一般的な表現］と［その語に特有の特徴］）が含まれ，定型表現として使われます．これらのパターンを学習すれば，新しい言葉の意味を早く正確に理解することができるばかりか，英文を書くときや，研究発表をするときなどにも役立ちます．

文法ノート：冠詞の役割

　　［定義する語］is/are （一般的な名詞）　＋　<u>具体的な特徴</u>

（　　）の中には名詞が入ります．名詞には冠詞が必要な場合があります．

- 冠詞の a が必要：数えられる名詞で同様のものがほかにもありえる（限定しない）とき
- 冠詞を入れない：数えられない名詞あるいは数えられる名詞の複数形で同様のものがほかにもありえる（限定しない）とき
- 冠詞の the が必要：特徴がその語にしか当てはまらない（限定する）とき

Ⅱ   Language focus

6   Sentence patterns： Defining matter or a concept

What is science？In order to answer this question, you need to supply the definition of the word, **science**, as shown in the example below.

> **Science** *is a system of knowledge about the universe, based primarily on observation and experimentation.*

In scientific English, the author often provides definitions of the terms he or she uses as keywords in the paper, so it is important to know how to read and write definitions efficiently.

In general, a verb and three pieces of information are used in definition sentences.

| Word to be defined | + | a defining verb | + | (a/the) general class | + | characteristics | .

1. the word to be defined： [   ]
2. a defining verb： _____
3. the general class the word belongs to： (   )
4. specific characteristics： _____ .

[Science] is a (system of knowledge) about the universe, based primarily on observation and experimentation.

Defining verbs include： concerns, denotes, describes, indicates, involves, is called, is known as, means, stands for

Sentence patterns

1a. [   ] **is** a/an/the/(∅) (   ) preposition + _____ .
1b. [   ] **is** a/an/the/(∅) (modifier +   ).
1c. [   ] **is** a/an/the/(∅) (   ) that _____ .
2.   [   ] **refers to** a/an/the/(∅) (   ) _____ .
3.   [   ] **is / may be defined as** a/an/the/(∅) (   ) _____ .

To clarify or explain scientific words writers can also use the following to indicate definitions：

- Restatement signals： i.e., or, that is
- Punctuations： parentheses, colons, commas, dashes, quotation marks

7 **Application: Using the sentence patterns**

Basic composition exercises

7 A Paraphrasing: Look at the terms in "4A Words in context." Use the information from the reading to write the definitions of the following terms. Use your own words.

mosquito

malaria

Anopheles gambiae

vector

Limburger cheese

Brevibacterium epidermidis

7 B Sentence completion: Fill in the blanks. Listen to the recording and check your answers. (1～5)

1. A metronome is (   ) (   ) (   ) marking time by means of regularly recurring ticks or flashes at adjustable intervals.

2. The broadfork is (   ) large, heavy (   ) (   ) (   ) cultivate and aerate soil in place.

3. Trans-palmitoleic acid (   ) (   ) fatty (   ) (   ) (   ) found in milk, cheese, yogurt, and butter.

◀)) Track 2

4. Wind shear (   ) to (   ) change in winds between the lower and upper atmosphere.

5. A waterspout (   ) (   ) by (   ) National Weather Service (   ) (   ) tornado over water.

7 C   Oral exercise： Listen to the recording and answer the questions.

1. _____

2. _____

🔊)) **Track 3**

3. _____

4. _____

5. _____

Advanced composition exercises

7 D   Work with your partner. Read the examples below and indicate each part of the definition, using the notation system in the box.

> 1. the word to be defined： [   ]
> 2. a defining verb： ＿＿＿＿＿
> 3. the general class the word belongs to： (   )
> 4. specific characteristics： ＿＿＿＿＿.

Example： [Asthma] is a chronic, generally reversible (disease) of the airways.

1. Elastic potential energy is energy stored as a result of applying a force to deform an elastic object.

2. Anemia is defined as a decrease in hemoglobin (or hematocrit) level from an individual's baseline value.

3. Mitochondria (singular： mitochondrion) are organelles within eukaryotic cells that produce adenosine triphosphate (ATP), the main energy molecule used by the cell.

4. Malaria is a parasitic disease that involves high fevers, shaking, chills, flu-like symptoms, and anemia.

5. Biochemistry is the branch of science that explores the chemical processes within and related to living organisms.

7 E   Paraphrase each sentence in 7D using your own words.

1. _____

   _____

2. _____

   _____

3. _____

   _____

4. _____

   _____

5. _____

   _____

　Homo sapiens ホモ・サピエンスが，私たち人類が所属する種の学名であることは知っていますね．それでは，*Prunus serrulata* は何の学名でしょう．春になるとピンク色の花を咲かせ，皆が集う場を提供してくれる桜のことです．身近な例を二つあげましたが，これらは世界共通の［二名法］(binomen/binomial name) という方法でつけられています．

　二名法とは生物の種の学名の付け方です．これは，分類学の父とよばれるスウェーデンの生物学者/植物学者でもあったカール・フォン・リンネが提唱し，確立したものです．生物の分類は，［界・門・綱・目・科・属・種］(Kingdom, Division, Class, Order, Family, Genus, Species) の順番で細かくなります．学名は，［属名(*Genus*)＋種名(*species*)］をラテン語でイタリック体を用いて表記されます．

　では，ホモ・サピエンスを例にしてみましょう．

Homo	*sapiens*
属名(*Genus*)	種名(*species*)
名詞	形容詞
最初の文字は大文字	最初の文字は小文字

同じテキスト中で2回目以降に出てきた場合は以下のように表記できます．

H.	*sapiens*
イニシャル使用可	イニシャル使用不可

Unit 1 の Reading にも学名がいくつかでてきました．たとえば，*Brevibacterium epidermidis* は，ブレビバクテリウム属エピデルミディス種ということを表し，*B. epidermidis* とも表記されます．

| III | **Vocabulary and vocabulary learning skills** |

8 Words in the reading text

8 A Classify the words according to their parts of speech. There may be no words for a part of speech.

☐ acid	☐ associate *something* with	☐ carboxylic	☐ comparable
☐ composition	☐ confirm	☐ distinctive	☐ carbon dioxide
☐ evidence	☐ exhale	☐ genus	☐ harness
☐ hypothesize	☐ itchy	☐ microorganism	☐ moist
☐ odor	☐ organism	☐ potential	☐ pungent
☐ species	☐ subsist	☐ synthetic	☐ transmit
☐ vector	☐ host		

Check the box ☑ when you have learned the word.

nouns	verbs	adjectives	adverbs
acid			

8 B Choose four nouns from above and write a definition for each.

[   ] _____

[   ] _____

[   ] _____

[   ] _____

8 C Discuss the terms above with your partner.

You: What does (   ) mean ?

Your partner: (   ) means _____ .

9 Word-formation: Prefixes related to numbers

Many scientific words contain prefixes that are related to numbers.

Examples:

- <u>uni</u>cellular organism vs. <u>multi</u>cellular organism
- carbon <u>di</u>oxide vs. carbon <u>mono</u>xide
- <u>octa</u>nol
- These data confirmed <u>pluri</u>potency of iPS-MEF10 and iPS-MEF4 and <u>nulli</u>potency of iPS-MEF3 *in vitro*.[3)]

9 A   Numerical prefixes: Choose the words from the box on the next page to fill in the blanks.

meaning	prefixes	examples
0	nulli-	( ), nullipotent, nullisomy
1/2	semi-, hemi-	seminar, ( )
1	uni-, prim-, mono-, prot-	unicellular, primitive, monosaccharide, ( )
2	du-, bi-, second-, di-, dy-, duo-	duplicate, ( ), secondary, dichotomy, dyad, duodenum
3	tri-, ter-	triphosphate, triplicate, trisomy, triangle, tertiary
4	quadru-, quarter-, tetra-, tetrakis-	quadruple, ( ), tetragon, tetrakisphosphate
5	quin-, quint-, penta-	quintuple, quintuplet, quintet, quintan fever, pentagon
6	sext-, hex-	sextuple, hexagon
7	sept-, hepta-	September, heptad, ( )
8	oct-, octo-	octamer, octagon, octanol, octopus, octane
9	novem-, nona-	November, nonamer, nonane
10	decem-, dec-, decim-, deca-	December, decade, decimal, decane, ( )
10^2	hecto-	hectometer, hectopascal
10^3	kilo-	kilogram, ( )
10^6	mega-	megahertz, megawatt
10^9	giga-	gigabyte, gigacycle
10^{12}	tera-	( ), teracycle
10^{-1}	deci-	( ), decimal point
10^{-2}	centi-	centimeter, ( )
10^{-3}	milli-	millimeter, milligram, ( )
10^{-6}	micro-	micrometer, microwave oven
10^{-9}	nano-	nanogram, ( )
10^{-12}	pico-	picogram
many	multi-, pluri-, poly-	polyphenol, multiplication
few	pauci-, oligo-	paucity, ( )
all	tot-	total, ( ), totality

biannual	centipede	decapoda	deciliter	hemisphere
heptagon	kilowatt	millisecond	nanomole	nullify
oligophagous	protozoa	quarterly	terabyte	totipotency

9 B Look at a scientific text (e.g., scientific journals, textbooks, scientific news articles, etc.) and find 10 words that contain one (or more) numerical prefixes in the table. Write them in the box below.

word	prefix	meaning	word	prefix	meaning
1.			6.		
2.			7.		
3.			8.		
4.			9.		
5.			10.		

9 C Underline the numerical prefixes introduced in this unit and write the Japanese equivalent for each of the following terms.

1. dicarboxylic acid (   )
2. quadriceps femoris (   )
3. duodenum (   )
4. tritium (   )
5. biennial plant (   )
6. monoclonal antibody (   )
7. pentose (   )
8. docosahexaenoic acid (   )
9. tetracycline (   )
10. tricuspid valve (   )

9 D Write the English compound name for each of the following molecular formulas.

1. CO (   )
2. SO_2 (   )
3. NO (   )
4. SiO_2 (   )

Ⅳ   Scientific communication

10   Academic organizations

科学コミュニケーション

科学コミュニケーションとは，［科学に関する情報の伝達と共有］です．それでは，この科学に関する情報を誰にどうやって伝達し，また誰とどこで共有するのでしょうか．

学会・学術誌

　学会とは研究者同士が学術情報の伝達や共有をするための組織／団体です．学会では，定期的に研究発表の場があり，口頭で他の研究者に向けて研究成果を発信し，共有します．さまざまな議論が研究者間で行われ，研究の質をより高め，洗練されたものにしていきます．

　学会は，研究者がおのおのの研究成果を論文にしたものを集め，学術誌として刊行する機能もあります．学術誌に掲載するに足る論文か否かは，同じ分野の研究者による査読というプロセスを経て決定します．学術誌に掲載された論文は，先行研究としてほかの研究者が行う研究に貢献します．

科学雑誌・科学新聞

　最新の科学情報，新しい技術の紹介，さまざまな調査や研究から得られた結果や成果，科学分野関連著作の書評などを扱う一般向け総合誌から，専門分野に特化したものまで幅広くあります．研究者や専門家は，科学雑誌や新聞を通じてより広く一般の人たちへ情報を伝達し，共有します．

---

11   Exercise   対応するものを結びなさい.

学術誌	・	・ academic conference
組織としての学会／研究会	・	・ academic journal
会議としての学会／研究会	・	・ academic paper
学術論文	・	・ academic organization
学位論文	・	・ book review
査読	・	・ dissertation
研究者	・	・ manuscript
先行研究	・	・ peer review
研究成果（科学分野の）	・	・ preceding study
（論文の）原稿	・	・ researcher/s
科学雑誌	・	・ scientific findings
書評	・	・ scientific magazine

Unit 2
Classifying and Giving Examples

For example, science is a ⋯

Unit 2 では以下の事柄を学びます.

I. Reading and listening

Topic 2　PCR: A Method for Solving Mysteries of History
"PCR で歴史の謎を解く"

1 Pre-reading activities

2 Reading text

3 Understanding the structure

4 Reading for details: Finding the examples in a text
文章から例示情報を見つける

5 Note-taking: Looking for the thesis statement and topic
sentences of a text
テキストの構成を理解する

II. Language focus

6 Sentence patterns: Classifying and giving examples
物や事柄を分類する・例示する

7 Application: Using the sentence patterns

III. Vocabulary and vocabulary learning skills

8 Words in the reading text

9 Word-formation: Affixes related to time, size, and location
語形成: 時, 大きさ, 場所に関連する接辞を学ぶ

IV. Scientific communication

10 Types of scientific publications
学術誌に掲載される著作物の種類を知る

11 Exercise

Workbook（Unit 2）▶ p. W13

I   Reading and listening

Topic 2   PCR： A Method for Solving Mysteries of History

1 Pre-reading activities

1 A   Discuss the following with your partner.

1. Have you ever heard of PCR?

2. What do you think the Russian Imperial Romanov family and King Tutankhamun have in common?

3. How long do you think a dead body can be preserved in a glacier?

1 B   Listening activities   (Track 4)

1. Listen to the recording and write the keywords from the text.

2. Listen again, paying attention to intonation, pronunciation, and pauses.

3. Read the text below aloud with the recording.

2 Reading text   (Track 4)

◀)) Track 4

Topic 2

PCR： A Method for Solving Mysteries of History

DNA is often called the blueprint of life. Reading the sequence of DNA allows you to see the characteristics of an animal. Your DNA analysis can tell you many things about yourself, for example, your risk of developing diseases, your biological relationships, and some researchers even say it can reveal your temperament. However, in order to identify a DNA segment, researchers need a number of copies of it. In the 1980s, a technique called the polymerase chain reaction (PCR), which makes multiple copies of a specific DNA segment using a simple procedure in a test tube, was developed. It made it possible for scientists to amplify and identify genes in a very short time. Since then, the PCR method has evolved and it can now be categorized into four types： standard PCR, hot-start PCR, high fidelity PCR and specialty PCR. Each type has its own applications. In general, PCR has been used in many areas of science including biology and medicine to study characteristics of organisms. Interestingly enough, it is not only science where PCR is used but also the field of history where it is used to solve mysteries of the past.

One example in which PCR was used is the identification of the remains of the Russian Imperial Romanov family. Soon after the Russian Revolution broke out, the Romanov family was taken prisoner by the armed forces and secretly executed in Yekaterinburg in 1918. The family doctor and three servants were also put to death, bringing the total number of those who were killed to eleven. After the collapse of the Soviet Union, scientists searched for the burial place of the family, and dug up the remains of nine people in 1991. To conclusively determine that the remains were of the Romanov family, the scientists used PCR. PCR was again used when the remains of the last two missing imperial family members were found in 2007. After two years of testing, in 2009, scientists declared that all the remains had been identified and there were no remaining survivors of the Romanov imperial family.

PCR was also used to investigate Ötzi, the iceman who was found in the Tirolean Alps in 1991. Ötzi is a natural mummy that was well preserved in a glacier for a long time. Carbon dating revealed that he died more than 5000 years ago. His possessions indicate that he was a wealthy man. CT scans and X-rays showed that he had been killed with an arrow. However, who he was genetically or if he is linked to any modern humans remained a mystery. To unravel this, scientists used PCR and found that he is an ancestor of modern Europeans who live in Austria. The genetic investigation even identified 19 living people who are related to Ötzi.

Another example of a long-unsolved mystery is that of King Tutankhamun's family, which would not have been solved without PCR. King Tutankhamun, known as King Tut, was a king of ancient Egypt who ruled in the 14th century BC. Following the discovery of King Tut's almost intact tomb in 1922, several X-ray examinations were conducted, revealing that he had a bone disease and died at the age of 19. However, his kinship was not determined until 2008, when scientists used PCR to analyze the mummy of King Tut and 10 other royal mummies. The results indicated that his parents were brother and sister, children of King Amenhotep III and his wife Tiye.

PCR has contributed to identifying many other remains including those of King Richard III of England (1452−1485), whose remains were found in 2012. This method is useful in that it can make a positive identification even with the smallest remains of an organism.

3 Understanding the structure

3 A Text analysis

1. Read the text once again and write the keywords from the text. Compare with the answers in "1 B Listening activities."

2. How many paragraphs are there？ There are （   ） paragraphs.

3. What mysteries of history have been solved by the use of PCR？
   （   ） paragraphs.

3 B Skimming

1. What is the main purpose of the text？

2. List all the examples of historical mysteries that were solved using the PCR method.

4 Reading for details： Finding the examples in a text

4 A Words in context

1. Underline the following terms in the text and match each with its definition in the box.

1	biological relationships	（ ）	a A part of DNA
2	identify	（ ）	b Continuing to exist
3	DNA segment	（ ）	c A method of calculating the age of extremely old objects by measuring the amount of a particular type of carbon in them
4	amplify genes	（ ）	d People who are genetically related to each other
5	application	（ ）	e The practical purpose for which a machine, idea, etc. can be used, or a situation when this is used
6	remains (n)	（ ）	f The body of someone who has died
7	remain (v)	（ ）	g To be left after other things have been dealt with
8	remaining (adj)	（ ）	h To produce multiple copies of a gene sequence
9	carbon dating	（ ）	i To recognize something or discover exactly what it is, what its nature or origin is, etc.

2. Write the Japanese translation for the following terms.

	English	Japanese
1	DNA segment	
2	amplify genes	
3	application	
4	carbon dating	
5	identify	

3. Highlight the expressions in the reading that either show exemplification or categorization.

4 B   Scanning： Where can you find the answers to the questions below？ Underline the parts in the text. Discuss the answers with your partner.

1. What is PCR？

2. What did scientists find out about Ötzi using carbon dating, CT scans and X-rays？

3. What did scientists use the PCR method for when examining King Tut's mummy？

4 C   Schematization and extension： Work in groups. Discuss the answers to the following questions.

1. The chart below describes when and how the remains of the Romanov Imperial family were identified. Fill in the missing information based on the text.

Event	Put a check mark (✓) if PCR was used.
( ) The Romanov family and others were killed in Yekaterinburg.	
1991	✓
2007	
( ) Scientists finally identified all the remains of the Russian Imperial Romanov family.	

2. How many people were there in the Romanov family?

There were (   ) people in the family.

3. Which example is the most interesting to you? Why?

4. Give examples of diseases that can be detected using PCR.

5. What other purposes is PCR used for?

5 Note-taking: Looking for the thesis statement and topic sentences of a text

5 A Read the **Study Guide** (p. 2) and learn about thesis statements. Which paragraph introduces the thesis statement?

5 B Write the thesis statement.

5 C Underline the topic sentence of each body paragraph.

文型ノート：例示を **example** で表すとき

　説明したり，説得するときに例を用いると説得力が増します．科学論文でも例示の表現は頻繁に使用されるので，文型を覚えるようにしましょう．例を示す身近な表現として，for example がありますが，論文でもよく使われます．For example は文頭でも，挿入句としても使えるので便利な表現ですが，example の名詞としての用法には注意が必要です．［例として］の英訳として as an example/as examples のような副詞的なフレーズがありますが冗長になるので，名詞で使うときは Examples include など主語として明確に書くほうがすっきりと伝わります．

文法ノート：分類に必要な事柄

　何かを分類するときに，必要な事柄としては，A＝分類するもの，B＝分類の基準，C＝下位分類があります．

　　　A is divided into C based on B.

　　　We classified A into C by/according to B.

基準を明確にすると理解しやすくなります．

Ⅱ   Language focus

6   Sentence patterns： Classifying and giving examples

Some people **classify** natural science **into** two main branches： life science and physical science. Physical science is further **divided into** four subfields： chemistry, physics, astronomy and earth sciences. In life science, there are several subfields **such as** botany, zoology and medicine.

Scientific analysis starts with classification. After classifying something into groups, scientists often give examples that belong to each group. So, it is important to know the sentence patterns used in classification and exemplification. In this unit, we will learn the sentence structures to describe classification and exemplification.

Classifying

In general, there are two sentence patterns to classify a concept.

(1) Using classification verbs (passive voice)：

> Concept + is a classification verb (p.p.) + into/as subdivisions .

Classification verbs： classify, group, divide, categorize, etc.
Example： (The cells) <u>were classified</u> into [three types].
(The cells) <u>were classified</u> as [non-spread], [half-spread], or [completely spread].

(2) Using classification nouns：

> There are + number + a classification noun (plural) + in concept .

Classification nouns： taxonomy, class, category, kind, type, group, list, etc.
Example： There are <u>five</u> 〈classes〉 in the vertebrates.

Sentence patterns

1. (Item to be classified) is <u>classified</u> into [subdivisions].
2. There are <u>number</u> 〈classification nouns〉.

Giving examples

The following three sentence patterns are often used to give examples.

(1) Using a linking phrase：

> Statement of a concept . + Linking phrase , + example/s .

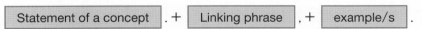

Linking phrases： For/for example, For/for instance, To/to illustrate, etc.

Example: [Some vegetables are high in vitamin C]. For example, (one cup of cooked broccoli has 101 mg of vitamin C).

(2) Using a be-verb:

| Example/s | + | be verb | + (an) example/examples of | concept. | .

Example: (Alzheimer's disease) is an example of [aging-associated diseases].

(3) Using adjectives (and others):

Examples are often inserted after a noun phrase.

| Concept | + | an exemplifying phrase | + | example/s | .

Exemplifying phrases: such as, including, like

Example: [Many animals] such as (dodo birds) and (California grizzly bears) have become extinct due to human activities.

Sentence patterns

1. [Statement of a concept]. For example, (examples).
2. (Example) is an example of [concept].
3. [Concept] such as (examples).

7　Application: Using the sentence patterns

Basic composition exercises

7 A　Paraphrasing: Use the information from the reading and write sentences following the directions. Use your own words.

1. Give examples of the things that your DNA analysis results can tell you.

```



```

2. Explain how today's PCR method is categorized.

```



```

3. Give examples of areas of science where PCR is used.

```



```

4. Give examples of mysteries of history that were solved by PCR.

7 B   Sentence completion: Fill in the blanks. Listen to the recording and check your answers.

1. Animals can be (   ) (   ) two main groups: vertebrates and invertebrates.
2. (   ) are 13 types of social media, (   ) blogs, business networks, forums, photo sharing, social gaming, and several more.
3. Synthetic fabrics are entirely made from chemicals. (   ) (   ), nylon and polyester are two common synthetic fabrics.
4. (   ) (   ) two (   ) within the genus *Panthera*: *Panthera leo* (lion) and *Panthera* onca (jaguar).
5. Entertainment (   ) be (   ) (   ) movies, TV programs, animations, and so on.

🔊) **Track 5**

7 C   Oral exercise: Listen to the recording and answer the questions.

1. _____
2. _____
3. _____
4. _____
5. _____

🔊) **Track 6**

Advanced composition exercises

7 D   Work with your partner. Read the examples below and indicate each part of the classification, using the notation system in the box.

1. concept to be classified: (   )
2. classification verb: ﹏﹏﹏
3. subdivisions: [   ]
4. classification number: _____
5. classification nouns: ⟨   ⟩

Example: The (cells) <u>were classified</u> as [non-spread], [half-spread], or [completely spread].

1. Polyurethane catalysts can be classified into two broad categories, amine compounds and organometallic complexes.
2. There are three major types of cell division: binary fission, mitosis, and meiosis.

7 E   Work with your partner. Read the examples below and indicate each part of the exemplification, using the notation system in the box.

---

1. statement of a concept or a concept/noun phrase to be exemplified: [   ]
2. linking phrase: ﹏﹏﹏﹏
3. examples: (   )
4. exemplifying phrase: _____.

Example: [A tablet] is a flat thin mobile computer. For example, two of the most popular tablets are (Apple's iPad) and (Samsung's Galaxy Tablet).

1. There are a number of factors that cause species to become endangered including human destruction of natural habitats and global warming.

2. Citrus fruits, such as oranges and grapefruits, are high in vitamin C.

3. Smoking can have many adverse effects on body systems. For example, the respiratory system, the circulatory system, and the reproductive system are all vulnerable to nicotine and other chemicals included in cigarettes.

7 F   Paraphrase each sentence above (Exercises 7 D and 7 E) using your own words.

(7 D) 1. _____

2. _____

(7 E) 1. _____

2. _____

3. _____

Ⅲ   Vocabulary and vocabulary learning skills

8   Words in the reading text

8 A   Write the part of speech for each word in the parentheses. Use these abbreviations:
noun = n   verb = v   adjective = adj   adverb = adv

☐ carbon dating ( )	☐ chain reaction ( )	☐ collapse ( )	☐ conclusively ( )
☐ conduct ( )	☐ contribute ( )	☐ execute ( )	☐ glacier ( )
☐ identify ( )	☐ imperial ( )	☐ indicate ( )	☐ intact ( )
☐ investigate ( )	☐ kinship ( )	☐ method ( )	☐ mummy ( )
☐ procedure ( )	☐ remains ( )	☐ reveal ( )	☐ revolution ( )
☐ segment ( )	☐ sequence ( )	☐ specific ( )	☐ survivor ( )
☐ temperament ( )	☐ unravel ( )	*Check the box* ☑ *when you have learned the word.*

8 B   Which words can be learned with the image strategy? Choose three and show how you use the strategy. You can use Japanese.

Example: chain reaction	*A reaction that occurs as a response to one change.* 鎖のように連続して起こる反応
1.	
2.	
3.	

8 C   Discuss the terms above with your partner.

You: What does (   ) mean?

Your partner: (   ) means _____ .

9 Word-formation: Affixes related to time, size and location

Many scientific words have affixes that are related to time and physical properties.

Examples:

- hypertension vs. hypotension
- pretest vs. posttest
- microscope vs. telescope

9 A Affixes related to physical properties: Choose the words from the box on the next page to fill in the blanks.

function	meaning	affixes	examples
time	after	post-	postnatal, postmortem, posterior
	back, again	re-	( ), reagent, reactor
	before	pre-, pro-, ante-	previously, proceed, antemortem
	circle, year	ann-, enni-	annual, ( )
	first	prim-, alpha-	( ), primer, *Alphaproteobacteria*
	time	chron-	chronic, chronoamperometry
size	half	hemi-, semi-, medi-, meso-	hemisphere, semiconductor, medium
	large	macro-, mega-, magn-	macrophage, ( )
	small	micro-, min-	microorganism, microscope
	small (amount)	oligo-	oligonucleotide, oligosaccharide
location	across	trans-, di-, dia-	transfer, diameter, diagonal
	alongside	para-	parameter, ( )
	away from	ab-	aberration, ablation
	away, not	dis-, dys-, im-, in-	disperse, dissociate, distillation
	before, front	ante-	anterior
	below, beneath	hypo-, sub-, infra-	( ), substrate, infrared
	between	inter-, medi-, mes-, meta-	interaction, ( ), mesophilic
	beyond	ultra-	ultrapure, ultraviolet, ultrasound
	center	nuc-, centr-	( ), nucleus, centrifuge
	high	alt-	altitude, altimeter
	outside, external	ecto-, ex-, exo-	ectodomain, extract, exoskeleton
	over, above	hyper-, super-	( ), hyperhydration
	place	-arium, loc-	aquarium, ( ), locus
	toward, to	ad-	adhere, ( ), adduct
	upon	epi-	( ), epidemic
	upward, apart	an-, dif-	diffuse, different
	with, together	co-, com-, syn-	( ), covalent, compose
	within	endo-, intra-	endosome, ( ), intracellular
	without	de-, e-, ex-, ef-, a-, an-	( ), extract, effluent, anhydrous

adjacent	biennial	coefficient	degrade	endogenous
epidermis	hyperbolic	hypoxia	locate	macromonomer
medium	nucleotide	parallel	primate	reaction

9 B   Look at a scientific text（e.g., scientific journals, textbooks, scientific news articles, etc.）and find 10 words that have one (or more) affixes related to time, size and location. Write them in the box below.

	word	affix	meaning		word	affix	meaning
1.				6.			
2.				7.			
3.				8.			
4.				9.			
5.				10.			

9 C   Underline the affixes introduced in this unit and write the Japanese equivalent for each of the following terms.

1. microbial component   ( )
2. posttest analysis   ( )
3. premature baby   ( )
4. hypercube   ( )
5. biannual   ( )
6. primatologist   ( )
7. episodic hypertension ( )
8. endocrine disruptor   ( )
9. deforestation   ( )
10. distilled water   ( )

9 D   Write the English equivalent for each of the following Japanese terms.

1. 内分泌系   ( )
2. 低血圧   ( )
3. （細胞の）中心体   ( )
4. 微生物学的検定   ( )

| **IV** | **Scientific communication** |

10   Types of scientific publications

学術誌に掲載される著作物の種類

科学コミュニケーションを行うにあたり，学会が発行する学術誌に掲載される著作物にはどのような種類のものがあるのでしょう？ここでは，どの分野にも共通する著作物のおもな種類を見ていきましょう.

原著論文

　一般に〈論文〉とよばれるものです. 著者（個人または研究チーム）の独自の視点に基づく研究を客観的かつ論理的に取りまとめたもの（研究背景および目的，研究手法，結果，考察および結論）を指します. 原著論文は出版物として未発表のものであり，相当の研究期間を費やした内容に基づくため，ページ数は学術誌に掲載される著作物の中では最も長いものになります. 原著論文が学術誌に掲載されることは，研究がその分野で認められたということを意味します.

総説論文

　すでに学術誌に掲載されている論文の内容に関して，要約，分析，その他研究との比較などを通して，今後の研究課題，発展のための提言をするものです. 自身が研究が研究しようと考えている分野やテーマに関する総説論文を読むと，これまでどのような事が明らかになってきたか，それに関する問題点，未解決事項などを把握することができます.

見解論文，意見論文，論評

　見解論文は，研究分野における基本概念や広く普及している考えに関して，著者個人の見解を学術的に述べるものです. 意見論文は，特定の研究や研究論文の有効性や課題に関して，著者の見解を述べるものです. 論評は，すでに出版されている論文，書籍または報告に関して，著者が興味を抱いた点などを簡潔に，かつ読者の注意を引くように書くものです. ページ数は上記2種類よりも短くまとめます.

プロシーディング

　学術会議（学会）で口頭発表するためには事前に発表したい内容の概略を主催する学術組織（学会）に提出します. 承認されると学会で発表する機会が与えられますが，それら概略を冊子としてまとめたものをプロシーディングとよびます.

11   Exercise

次の日本語に相当する英語を調べて書きなさい.

原著論文 _____

総説論文 _____

プロシーディング _____

速報 _____

修士論文 _____

博士論文 _____

Unit 3
Cause and Effect
Smoking causes …

Unit 3 では以下の事柄を学びます.

I. Reading and listening

Topic 3　Research Article Abstracts
　　　　"研究論文の抄録を読む"

1 Pre-reading activities

2 Reading text

3 Understanding the structure

4 Reading for details： Understanding cause and effect
原因と結果を理解する

5 Note-taking： Main ideas and details
抄録のポイントをつかむ

II. Language focus

6 Sentence patterns： Describing causal relationships
物や事柄の原因とその影響を表現する

7 Application： Using the sentence patterns

III. Vocabulary and vocabulary learning skills

8 Words in the reading text

9 Word-formation： Negative/positive and paired affixes
反意の接辞，対になる接辞，品詞をつくる接辞を学ぶ

IV. Scientific communication

10 Structure of a research article： The abstract
IMRaD 論文の構成： 抄録について知る

11 Exercise

Workbook（Unit 3）▶ p. W 23

I   Reading and listening

Topic 3   Research Article Abstracts

1   Pre-reading activities

1 A   Read Scientific communications on p. 54 and learn about research article abstracts. Discuss the following with your partner.

1. What is a research article abstract?
2. What is the purpose of an abstract?

1 B   Listening activities   (Track 7)

1. Listen to the recording and write the keywords from the texts.

Abstract 1

Abstract 2

2. Listen again, paying attention to intonation, pronunciation, and pauses.

3. Read the text below aloud with the recording.

2   Reading text   (Track 7)

◀)) Track 7

Topic 3   Abstract 1

Thirdhand Cigarette Smoke: Factors Affecting Exposure and Remediation[4]

Abstract

Thirdhand smoke (THS) refers to components of secondhand smoke that stick to indoor surfaces and persist in the environment. Little is known about exposure levels and possible remediation measures to reduce potential exposure in contaminated areas. This study deals with the effect of aging on THS components and evaluates possible exposure levels and remediation measures. We investigated the concentration of nicotine, five nicotine related alkaloids, and three tobacco specific nitrosamines (TSNAs) in smoke exposed fabrics. Two different extraction methods were used. Cotton terry cloth and polyester fleece were exposed to smoke in controlled laboratory conditions and aged before extraction. Liquid chromatography-tandem mass spectrometry was used for chemical analysis. Fabrics aged for 19 months after smoke exposure retained significant amounts of THS chemicals. During aqueous extraction, cotton cloth released about 41 times as much nicotine and about 78 times the amount of tobacco specific nitrosamines (TSNAs) as polyester after one hour of aqueous extraction. Concentrations of nicotine and TSNAs in extracts of terry cloth exposed to smoke were used to estimate infant/ toddler oral exposure and adult dermal exposure to THS. Nicotine exposure from THS residue can be 6.8 times higher in toddlers and 24 times higher in adults and TSNA exposure can be 16 times higher in toddlers and 56 times higher in adults than what would be inhaled by a passive smoker. In addition to providing exposure estimates, our data could be useful in developing remediation strategies and in framing public health policies for indoor environments with THS.

Topic 3   Abstract 2

Water-Induced Finger Wrinkles Do Not Affect Touch Acuity or Dexterity in Handling Wet Objects[5)]

Abstract

Human non-hairy (glabrous) skin of the fingers, palms and soles wrinkles after prolonged exposure to water. Wrinkling is a sympathetic nervous system-dependent process but little is known about the physiology and potential functions of water-induced skin wrinkling. Here we investigated the idea that wrinkling might improve handling of wet objects by measuring the performance of a large cohort of human subjects ($n=40$) in a manual dexterity task. We also tested the idea that skin wrinkling has an impact on tactile acuity or vibrotactile sensation using two independent sensory tasks. We found that skin wrinkling did not improve dexterity in handling wet objects nor did it affect any aspect of touch sensitivity measured. Thus water-induced wrinkling appears to have no significant impact on tactile driven performance or dexterity in handling wet or dry objects.

3 Understanding the structure

3 A Text analysis

Abstracts in general consist of several parts: (1) the background of the study, (2) the objectives, (3) the methods used, (4) the results (numerical data) and (5) the discussion (including findings and sometimes usage of the findings). Read abstracts 1 and 2 and discuss the following.

1. Abstract 1 consists of [   ] parts which are_____.

2. Abstract 2 consists of [   ] parts which are_____.

3 B Skimming

Mark each part you found in "3 A Text analysis" in each abstract using highlighters.

4 Reading for details: Understanding cause and effect

4 A Words in context

1. Find and circle the following terms in the texts.

2. Based on the reading, explain each of the following terms in the boxes below.

Abstract 1

THS

| |
| |

THS chemicals

| |
| |

TSNAs

| |
| |

oral/dermal exposure

| |
| |

Abstract 2

glabrous skin

water-induced wrinkling

tactile acuity

a manual dexterity task

4 B   Scanning : Where can you find the answers to the questions below ? Underline the parts in the text. Discuss the answers with your partner.

Abstract 1

1. What is the cause of the problem ?
2. What kinds of fabric were used for the investigation ?
3. What experimental procedures were used in the study ?

Abstract 2

1. When does the skin of your fingers, palms and soles get wrinkled ?
2. How many people participated in the experiment ?
3. What did they measure ?
4. What results did they obtain ?

4 C   Schematization and extension : Work in groups. Discuss the answers to the following questions.

1. Do you think it is easy to handle wet objects when your fingers are wrinkled ?

2. Identify the events or things that have a cause-and-effect relationship in each abstract.

Example : smoking in a closed environment   ⟶   thirdhand smoke

Abstract 1 [   ] → [   ]

Abstract 2 [   ] → [   ]

4 D Verb tenses used in abstracts： Work in groups. Look for the examples in the two abstracts. Fill in the blanks.

	[Verb tense]	Usage	Abst. #	Examples from the two abstracts
Background	[Present]	Defining key terms/ notions	#1	Thirdhand smoke（THS）( ) ( ) components of secondhand smoke that stick to indoor surfaces and persist in the environment.
			#2	Wrinkling ( ) a sympathetic nervous system-dependent process but …
	[Present]	What is known about the topic	#1	( ) ( ) ( ) about exposure levels and possible remediation measures to reduce potential exposure in contaminated areas.
	[Present perfect]	Referring to previous studies	—	—
Objectives	[Present]	Introducing objectives of the study	#1	This study ( ) ( ) the effect of aging on THS components and evaluates possible exposure levels and remediation measures.
	[Past]	Introducing what the researchers did	#2	( ) we ( ) the idea that wrinkling might improve handling of wet objects …
Methodology	[Past]	Explaining how they carried out the research	#1	Two different extraction ( ) ( ) ( ).
Results	[Past]	Telling the results	#2	We ( ) ( ) skin wrinkling did not improve dexterity in handling wet objects nor did it affect any aspect of touch sensitivity measured.
Discussion	[Present]	Discussing the results	#2	Thus water-induced wrinkling ( ) ( ) have no significant impact on tactile drive performance or dexterity in handling wet or dry objects.

5 Note-taking： Main ideas and details

5 A Summarize the main ideas（findings）of the research in your own words.

Abstract 1

```
┌─────────────────────────────────────────────────────────┐
│                                                         │
│                                                         │
│                                                         │
└─────────────────────────────────────────────────────────┘
```

Abstract 2

```
┌─────────────────────────────────────────────────────────┐
│                                                         │
│                                                         │
│                                                         │
└─────────────────────────────────────────────────────────┘
```

5 B Review the background, objectives, methods and results of each abstract. Discuss with your partner how these sections（details）support the main ideas above.

文型ノート： 論文タイトル

　科学論文のタイトルには研究で扱ったものや事柄の因果関係を表した表現がよく使われます．論文で取扱っている因果関係を的確に表した一文をそのままタイトルにしているものが多く見られます．以下の二つの例は実際に出版された論文のタイトルですが，分野を問わずよく使われることがわかります．

例：

1. Arctic amplification **is caused by** sea-ice loss under increasing CO_2.[6]
2. Hereditary parkinsonism with dementia **is caused by** mutations in ATP13A2, encoding a lysosomal type 5 P-type ATP-ase.[7]

文法ノート： Hedges（ぼかし表現）　科学論文では物事の因果関係を表現することが多くあります．因果関係を証明することが，論文のテーマの場合もあります．そのため，因果関係を表すさまざまな表現がありますが，因果関係を 100 % 完全に証明できないことも多くあります．そのようなときに hedge とよばれるぼかし表現を使います．よく使われるものとしては **may, might, can, could** などの法助動詞，**seem, tend to, believe, suggest, indicate, appear to be** などの動詞，**probably, possibly, perhaps** などの副詞，**probable, possible** などの形容詞があります．論文中に hedges がどのように使用されているか確認しながら読んでいくと，だんだん使えるようになるものです．ぜひ，試してみましょう．

II   Language focus

6   Sentence patterns： Describing causal relationships

A new study reports Alzheimer's disease **may be caused by** bacteria in the brain.

In scientific writing, we need to state the relationship between the cause and its results. Several sentence patterns are used to show a causal relationship.

(1)   Using verbs

Three types of information are needed： [the cause], a verb, and (the results).

Causal verbs include： cause, create, contribute to, enable, lead to, result in, stem from, give rise to, affect, shape, increase, prevent, influence, determine, associate with, differentiate into, derive from, etc.

(**active**)

The cause + (may / can) + a causal verb + the results .

Example： [Deforestation] may cause (global warming).

(**passive**)

The results + be + a causal verb (p.p.) + by + the cause .

Example： (Global warming) is caused by [human activities such as burning fossil fuels, and farming].

(2)   Using linking phrases

Statement of the cause + a linking phrase + a statement of the results .

Phrases that indicate a causal relationship include： therefore, consequently, because, because of this, as a result, despite, in order to, due to, for this reason, etc.

Other expressions include： owing to, thus, thereby, etc.

Sentence patterns [the cause] (the result)

1. [   ] verb (   ).

2. [   ] may verb (   ).

3. (   ) is/are verb (p.p.) by [   ].

4. [   ]. As a result, (   ).

7   Application： Using the sentence patterns

Basic composition exercises

7 A   Paraphrasing： Use the information from the reading to describe the causal relationships related to the following events or things. Use your own words.

Abstract 1

THS

oral exposure

fabrics

Abstract 2

wrinkling

a/the manual dexterity task

tactile acuity

7 B   Sentence completion： Fill in the blanks. Listen to the recording and check your answers.   (1～5)

1. The gravitational pull of the moon and the sun (   ) high tide and low tide.

2. Infections can (   ) (   ) serious health problems.

3. Young people's opinions (   ) often (   ) (   ) messages and images on social media.

4. The flood water was dirty. (   ) (   ) (   ), many epidemics occurred.

◀)) Track 8

5. Cancer and cardiovascular disease share common risk factors. (   ), cancer patients are advised to eat healthily and exercise.

7 C Oral exercise: Listen to the recording and answer the questions.

🔊) Track 9

1. _____

2. _____

3. _____

4. _____

5. _____

Advanced composition exercises

7 D Work with your partner. Read the examples below and indicate each part of the causal relationship, using the notation system in the box.

> cause: [   ]
> phrase to indicate causal relationship: ~~~~~~~~~
> result: (   )

Example: [Asthma] is caused by (an inflammation of the airways).

1. These imported cases might result in local spread of the virus.
2. Histological analyses confirmed that iPS cells contributed to all three germ layers.[3]
3. Depression is likely to be due to a complex combination of factors.
4. Circulating monocytes give rise to mature macrophages.

7 E Paraphrase each sentence in 7 D using your own words.

1. _____

2. _____

3. _____

4. _____

| Ⅲ | **Vocabulary and vocabulary learning skills** |

8   Words in the reading text

8 A   Write the part of speech for each word in the parentheses. Use these abbreviations：
noun ＝ n   verb ＝ v   adjective ＝ adj   adverb ＝ adv

☐ acuity ( )	☐ component ( )	☐ concentration ( )	☐ contaminate ( )
☐ dermal ( )	☐ dexterity ( )	☐ exposure ( )	☐ extraction ( )
☐ impact ( )	☐ inhale ( )	☐ manual ( )	☐ palm ( )
☐ persist ( )	☐ physiology ( )	☐ prolonged ( )	☐ remediation ( )
☐ residue ( )	☐ retain ( )	☐ sensation ( )	☐ sensory ( )
☐ sole ( )	☐ significant ( )	☐ tactile ( )	☐ toddler ( )
☐ wrinkle ( )		*Check the box ☑ when you have learned the word.*	

8 B   Which words do you think are suitable to learn with the association strategy？
Choose three and show how you use the strategy. You can use Japanese.

例	toddler	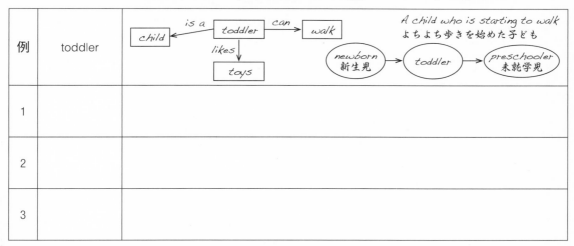
1		
2		
3		

8 C   Discuss the terms above with your partner.

You： What does (   ) mean？

Your partner： (   ) means _____.

9   Word-formation： Negative/positive and paired affixes

A lot of affixes are used to negate the meaning of the original word and knowing those affixes may significantly increase your vocabulary.

Examples:

- function ←→ <u>mal</u>function   · care<u>ful</u> ←→ care<u>less</u>   · <u>in</u>valid ←→ invalid

9 A   Affixes that change the meaning of the original word: Choose the words from the box on the next page to fill in the blanks.

meaning	affixes	examples
negate the original meaning	a-, an- anti- contra- counter- dis-, dys- ex-, e- false-, faux- in-, il-, im-, ir- ig- mal- neg- non- pseudo- quasi- un- -less	( ), asymptomatic antiseptic, ( ), antigen ( ), contrary counterview, counterstain dystrophy, ( ), dysfunction, dislocation exchange false-positive innocuous, ( ), insane ignoble, ignore malignant, malaria, ( ) negligible, negate, negative nonabrasive, nonfat pseudopodia, pseudoscience, pseudonym quasi drugs, ( ) undo, unanalyzable, unaltered ( ), leafless, motionless
pairs	bene- / mal- eu- / dys- exo- / endo- homo- / hetero- inter- / intra- paleo- / neo- -ful / -less	( ) / malignant eupepsia / dyspepsia exocrine / ( ) homogenous / heterogenous intercellular / ( ) paleolithic / neolithic useful / useless
change the part of speech	en- -ed -ful -ly -ous -some (cf., some=the body) -fy	enable, enlarge, encode deionized, ( ), infrared, sonicated careful, powerful, useful, unsuccessful respectively, previously, ( ) ( ), anomalous, amorphous troublesome purify, modify, ( ), identify

anaerobic	antibody	aqueous	benign	contradiction
degassed	disease	endocrine	flawless	intracellular
invalid	malnutrition	quantify	quasicrystal	subsequently

9 B Look at a scientific text (e.g., scientific journals, textbooks, scientific news articles, etc.) and find 10 words that contain one (or more) affixes introduced in this unit. Write them in the box below.

	word	affix	meaning		word	affix	meaning
1.				6.			
2.				7.			
3.				8.			
4.				9.			
5.				10.			

9 C Underline the affixes introduced in this unit and write the Japanese equivalent for each of the following terms.

1. quasi-linear equation   (   )
2. muscular dystrophy   (   )
3. pseudopod   (   )
4. dysentery   (   )
5. left unexposed   (   )
6. eupnea vs. dyspnea   (   )
7. intra-abdominal adhesion   (   )
8. asymmetric carbon atom   (   )
9. homogeneous and isotropic   (   )
10. antigen-binding domain   (   )

9 D Write the English equivalent for each of the following Japanese terms.

1. 栄養不良患者   (   )
2. 負の電荷を帯びたイオン   (   )
3. 脱気水   (   )
4. 屋内/屋外   (   )

Ⅳ   **Scientific communication**

🔟 Structure of a research article： The abstract

科学コミュニケーション

科学コミュニーケーションおいて，著作物／出版物は科学知識の構築，科学技術・研究の発展，科学教育に大きく貢献します．また，研究活動の成果として原著論文を執筆することは，研究者の使命ともいえます．それでは，研究活動の成果は実際にどのように論文としてまとめるのでしょう？ここからは論文の構成とそのセクションを順番に説明します．

論文の構成
　論文の構成は各学会や学術誌により若干の規定の違いはありますが，次のような共通のセクションがあります：論文題目，抄録，序論，方法，結果，考察，参考文献，謝辞

抄録／アブスト（abstract）
抄録とは何か
　上記序論から考察までを要約したもので，論文のセクションの一つですが独立したものです．抄録を読めば，詳細な研究方法や結果を読まなくても，論文の全体像を把握することができます．読み手の立場からは，抄録を読むことで，その研究が自身の研究の参考文献になるかどうかを判断することができます．

抄録の種類
　論文の種類は大きく分けて二つあります：説明型（descriptive）と情報提供型（informative）です．科学論文では，情報提供型を用います．この情報型は，さらに二つのタイプに分かれます：構造化（structured）と非構造化（unstructured）です．構造化抄録を書く場合は，前出のセクションの見出しのもと，各セクションを要約します．非構造化抄録は，論文の内容を一つのパラグラフに要約します．抄録のスタイルは学術誌によって異なるので，研究者は論文を投稿する学術誌の規定に従って書く必要があります．

🔢 Exercise

次の日本語に相当する英語を調べて書きなさい．

論文題目＿＿＿＿＿＿＿＿＿＿＿＿　　方　法　＿＿＿＿＿＿＿＿＿＿＿＿

抄　録　＿＿＿＿＿＿＿＿＿＿＿＿　　結　果　＿＿＿＿＿＿＿＿＿＿＿＿

序　論　＿＿＿＿＿＿＿＿＿＿＿＿　　考　察　＿＿＿＿＿＿＿＿＿＿＿＿

背　景　＿＿＿＿＿＿＿＿＿＿＿＿　　参考文献＿＿＿＿＿＿＿＿＿＿＿＿

目　的　＿＿＿＿＿＿＿＿＿＿＿＿　　謝　辞　＿＿＿＿＿＿＿＿＿＿＿＿

Unit 4
Purpose and Process
Two pathways lead to …

Unit 4 では以下の事柄を学びます.

I. Reading and listening

Topic 4　Introduction to Blood Coagulation
"血液凝固"

1 Pre-reading activities

2 Reading text

3 Understanding the structure

4 Reading for details： Understanding the purpose and the process／procedure in a text
文章中に示された目的と過程や手順の情報を見つける

5 Note-taking： Taking notes using Cornell style
コーネルスタイルを使ってノートを取る

II. Language focus

6 Sentence patterns： Describing the purpose and the process／procedure
目的・手順・変化の過程を述べる

7 Application： Using the sentence patterns

III. Vocabulary and vocabulary learning skills

8 Words in the reading text

9 Word-formation： Affixes related to chemistry
語形成： 化学でよく使われる接辞を学ぶ

IV. Scientific communication

10 Structure of a research article： The introduction
IMRaD 論文の構成： 序論について知る

11 Exercise

Workbook（Unit 4）▶ p. W 33

I   Reading and listening

Topic 4   **Introduction to Blood Coagulation**

1   Pre-reading activities

1 A   Discuss the following with your partner.

1. When you have a cut, how do you stop the bleeding?

2. Name a component of blood that helps your body form a clot to stop the bleeding.

3. Which protein in blood plasma is involved in the clotting of blood?

1 B   Listening activities   (Track 10)

1. Listen to the recording and write the keywords from the text.

2. Listen again, paying attention to intonation, pronunciation, and pauses.

3. Read the text below aloud with the recording.

2   Reading text   (Track 10)

◀)) **Track 10**

Topic 4

Introduction to Blood Coagulation

The ability of the body to control the flow of blood following vascular injury is paramount to continued survival. The process of blood clotting and then the subsequent dissolution of the clot, following repair of the injured tissue, is termed **hemostasis**. Hemostasis comprises four major events that occur in a set order following the loss of vascular integrity:

1. The initial phase of the process is vascular constriction. This limits the flow of blood to the area of injury.

2. Next, platelets become activated by **thrombin** and aggregate at the site of injury, forming a temporary, loose platelet plug. The protein fibrinogen is primarily responsible for stimulating platelet clumping. Platelets clump by binding to collagen that becomes exposed following rupture of the endothelial lining of vessels. Upon activation, platelets release the nucleotide,

ADP, and the eicosanoid, TXA_2 (both of which activate additional platelets), serotonin, phospholipids, lipoproteins, and other proteins important for the coagulation cascade. In addition to induced secretion, activated platelets change their shape to accommodate the formation of the plug.

3. To ensure stability of the initially loose platelet plug, a fibrin mesh (also called the **clot**) forms and entraps the plug. If the plug contains only platelets it is termed a **white thrombus**; if red blood cells are present it is called a **red thrombus**.

4. Finally, the clot must be dissolved in order for normal blood flow to resume following tissue repair. The dissolution of the clot occurs through the action of **plasmin**.

Two pathways lead to the formation of a fibrin clot: the intrinsic and extrinsic pathways. Although they are initiated by distinct mechanisms, the two converge on a common pathway that leads to clot formation. Both pathways are complex and involve numerous different proteins termed clotting factors. Fibrin clot formation in response to tissue injury is the most clinically relevant event of hemostasis under normal physiological conditions. This process is the result of the activation of the extrinsic pathway. The formation of a red thrombus or a clot in response to an abnormal vessel wall in the absence of tissue injury is the result of the intrinsic pathway. The intrinsic pathway has low significance under normal physiological conditions. Most significant clinically is the activation of the intrinsic pathway by contact of the vessel wall with lipoprotein particles, VLDLs and chylomicrons. This process clearly demonstrates the role of hyperlipidemia in the generation of atherosclerosis. The intrinsic pathway can also be activated by vessel wall contact with bacteria.

引用元 © 1996-2020 themedicalbiochemistrypage, LLC

3   Understanding the structure

3 A   Text analysis

1. Read the text once again and write the keywords from the text. Compare with the answers in "1 B Listening activities."

2. How many blood clotting events occur for a stable blood clot to be formed? In order for a stable blood clot to be formed, [   ] events need to occur.

3. Divide the second paragraph into three parts: the introduction of the two pathways, the intrinsic pathway, and the extrinsic pathway.

3 B   Skimming

1. What is the main purpose of the text?

2. What are the themes of the two paragraphs?

Paragraph 1

Paragraph 2

4   **Reading for details: Understanding the purpose and the process/procedure in a text**

4 A   Words in context

1. Use definition language (see Unit 1. Ⅱ) and define the following terms based on the information given in the text.

	Term	Definition
1	hemostasis	Hemostasis is the process of …
2	fibrinogen	Fibrinogen is a _____ which …
3	red thrombus	

2. Look at the underlined words in the following sentences. In which of the choices from "a" to "c" does the *italicized* word/phrase have **the same meaning** as the underlined part? Make sure you learn the Japanese translation of the word/phrase.

(1)   Next, platelets become underlined{activated} by thrombin and aggregate at the site of injury, forming a temporary, loose platelet plug.

a. Press the button to *activate* the system.

b. The alarm is *activated* when it senses smoke.

c. You need slightly warm water to *activate* yeast.

(2)   Most significant clinically is the activation of the intrinsic pathway by underlined{contact} of the vessel wall with lipoprotein particles, VLDLs and chylomicrons.

a. After he moved to France, I lost *contact* with him.

b. Through the project, students came in *contact* with people from different cultures.

c. Some people are allergic to rubbing alcohol. Symptoms occur in areas in *contact* with the substance.

(3) This process clearly demonstrates the role of hyperlipidemia in the <u>generation</u> of atherosclerosis.

a. We need to preserve nature for future *generations*.

b. SNSs are a popular way of connecting with other people among the younger *generations*.

c. Electricity is partly *generated* using renewable resources.

3. Underline the expressions that signal a process in the text.

Example : The initial phase of the process is vascular constriction.

4 B　Scanning : Where can you find the answers to the questions below ? Underline the parts in the text. Discuss the answers with your partner.

1. Of the four events in hemostasis, which refer to blood clotting ?

2. Read the second event in hemostasis. Underline the parts that describe thrombin and fibrinogen.

3. According to the text, the intrinsic pathway can be activated in response to any one of three events. What are they ?

4 C　Schematization and extension : Work in groups. Discuss the answers to the following questions.

1. The following graphics illustrate the process of blood clotting. Fill in the blanks with the appropriate phrase from the box below.

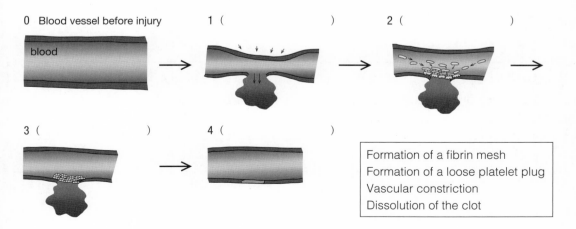

0　Blood vessel before injury　　　1 (　　　　　　)　　2 (　　　　　　)

blood

3 (　　　　)　　　4 (　　　　)

| Formation of a fibrin mesh |
| Formation of a loose platelet plug |
| Vascular constriction |
| Dissolution of the clot |

2. Write at least three things you do in the morning before leaving for school. List them in the order you do them.

1

2

3

4

5

文型ノート: 文中に示された目的を見つけながら methods を理解しよう

　Method のセクションでは，具体的な実験器具や方法が示されます．論文の情報から再現実験ができることが重要なので，論文には具体的で詳細な情報を載せています．多くの場合，その分野の研究者以外には馴染みのない名詞が並ぶため，読み解くのが難しく感じられます．ただ，実験器具や試薬がわからなくても，その手順の目的と結果が読み取れれば，論文の概要がわかります．実際の手順が書かれている部分を読むときは，そのプロセスの目的と得られる結果を示す英語表現に注目しましょう．

文法ノート: 論文の時制

　論文はセクションごとに使用される時制が変わります．Introduction と discussion には，現在形，現在完了形が多く使われ，methods と results では，過去形が多く使われます．特に，実際に行った実験について報告する methods のセクションでは，過去形の受動態が使われている文がほとんどであることを実際の論文を読みながら確認してみましょう．

5 Note-taking: Taking notes using Cornell style

Read the **Study Guide** (p. 3) and learn about Cornell notes. Then, complete the notes below.

What is hemostasis?	Hemostasis: The process of blood (　　　) and then the subsequent (　　　) of the clot, following repair of the injured tissue.
What happens in hemostasis?	1. Vascular constriction occurs. 2. Platelets activated by (　　　) aggregate at the site of injury and form a temporary, loose (　　　) (　　　). 3. A (　　　) mesh (clot) is formed to (　　　) the stability of the platelet plug. 4. Clot (　　　).
What two pathways lead to the formation of a fibrin clot?	(　　　) and (　　　) pathways lead to the formation of a fibrin clot.
What causes the extrinsic pathway to be (　　　)?	Tissue injury of the vessel wall causes _____ _____.
What is the result of the activation of the extrinsic pathway?	Fibrin (　　　) formation is _____ _____.
What causes the intrinsic pathway to be activated?	Abnormal vessel wall caused by the contact of the vessel wall with: 1. (　　　) particles 2. (　　　)
What is the result of the activation of the intrinsic pathway?	The formation of a red (　　　) or a clot

There are (number　　　) major events that occur in a fixed (　　　) in (　　　).
The intrinsic pathway, due to abnormal tissue, and the extrinsic pathway, caused by
(　　　) (　　　), lead to (　　　) (　　　) formation.

II	**Language focus**

6 Sentence patterns： Describing the purpose and the process/ procedure

Understanding the research method is not very difficult if you know the purpose and the expected results. The methods section contains information that states the purpose of the research and the process used in the experiment. The process is described using phrases that signal the sequence (sequence phrases) of procedures. These phrases are also used to describe naturally occurring processes as in the reading text in this unit.

Example：

To perform immunohistochemical analysis, muscles were mounted in tragacanth gum and frozen following different protocols.

(**purpose**) To perform immunohistochemical analyses, (**1st procedure**) muscles were mounted in tragacanth gum and (**2nd procedure**) frozen following different protocols.[8]

(1) The purpose of a procedure can be indicated by：

to	+	verb + phrase

for	+	(specific description) + noun

(2) The process of the study is often signaled by sequence words such as **first, second, third**, and many other expressions shown below.

A sequence phrase	+	a procedure	+	a second procedure	.

Before a procedure： prior to, before

At the beginning of a procedure： on, when

At the end of a procedure： at the end of

After a procedure： after, once, following

(3) The sequence can also be signaled by a sequence phrase as below.

A procedure	+	a sequence phrase	+	a second procedure	.

Actions performed after an action： then, next, and then, after that, subsequently, followed by, afterwards

Other words that often signal sequences: initially, then (adverb), subsequent (adjective), until (prep.)

1. purpose: _____

2. sequence phrase: (   )

3. procedure 1: ₁~~~~~~~~

4. procedure 2: ₂~~~~~~~~

Example:

In order to see if echinacea tea is effective as a treatment for a cold, ₁we called for volunteers who were diagnosed with a common cold. ₂These volunteers were (then) divided into two groups: one taking echinacea tea and the other taking a placebo.

7 Application: Using the sentence patterns

Basic composition exercises

7 A Use the information from the reading and complete the text to describe the following graphics. Use your own words.

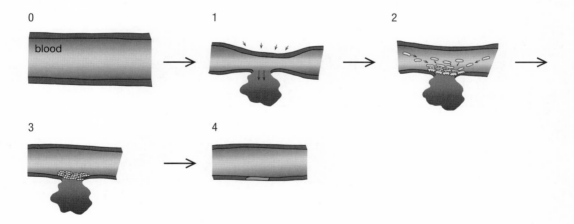

> The blood coagulation process can be explained as follows:

7 B   Sentence completion: Fill in the blanks. Listen to the recording and check your answers.

| after   before   to   once   subsequently |

Use one for each (   ).

🔊) Track 11

1. (   ) [identify   ] whose remains it was, researchers used the PCR method.

2. (   ) [remove   ] the tumor, a portion was sent to pathology for examination.

3. (   ) the cells [be   ] analyzed, researchers will have a better understanding of the mechanism.

4. (   ) mitosis [happen   ], a cell must make a second set of chromosomes.

5. The cells were (   ) washed three times and resuspended in culture medium.

7 C   Oral exercise: Listen to the recording and answer the questions.

🔊) Track 12

1. _____

_____

2. _____

_____

3. _____

_____

4. _____

_____

5. _____

_____

Advanced composition exercises

7 D Work with your partner. Read the text below and indicate each part of the description of the purpose and the process/procedure, using the notation system in the box.

---

1. purpose: _____
2. sequence phrase: (   )
3. procedure 1: 1_____
4. procedure 2: 2_____

The purpose of this experiment is to make dirty 10-yen coins look new again. For this experiment you will need the following items: dirty copper coins, vinegar, a non-metal bowl, water, paper towel.

First, put 50 ml of vinegar and 1 teaspoon of salt in a non-metal bowl. After that, stir until the salt is dissolved. Next, put two or three dirty 10-yen coins in the bowl for about 30 seconds. Then, take the coins out and rinse them with water. Finally, place the coins on a piece of paper towel to dry.

Once the coins are dry, you will have shiny coins which look like they were just made.

7 E Rewrite the text in 7D using your own words.

Ⅲ   Vocabulary and vocabulary learning skills

8   Words in the reading text

8 A   Write the part of speech for each word in the parentheses. Use these abbreviations :
noun ＝ n   verb ＝ v   adjective ＝ adj   adverb ＝ adv

☐ accommodate ( )	☐ activate ( )	☐ aggregate ( )	☐ cascade ( )
☐ clot ( )	☐ coagulation ( )	☐ comprise ( )	☐ constriction ( )
☐ dissolution ( )	☐ distinct ( )	☐ entrap ( )	☐ hemostasis ( )
☐ induce ( )	☐ integrity ( )	☐ lining ( )	☐ paramount ( )
☐ phase ( )	☐ platelet ( )	☐ plug ( )	☐ protein ( )
☐ resume ( )	☐ rupture ( )	☐ secretion ( )	☐ stability ( )
☐ subsequent ( )	☐ temporary ( )	☐ tissue ( )	☐ vascular ( )
☐ vessel ( )			

Check the box ☑ when you have learned the word.

8 B   Learn the words using the composition strategy. Give five examples below.

Example : induce	Like pollens and foods, stress can induce allergies.
1.	
2.	
3.	
4.	
5.	

8 C   Discuss the terms above with your partner.

You : What does (   ) mean ?

Your partner : (   ) means _____ .

9   Word-formation： Affixes related to chemistry

Many words in chemistry are related to actions and qualities （chloric … chloride）.

9 A   Affixes related to chemistry： Choose the words from the box on the next page to fill in the blanks.

function	meaning	affixes	examples
prefixes action	move	ag-, act-	agent, reagent, （ ）
	burn, heat	cau-, caus-	cauldron, cauterize
	lead, pull	duc-, duct-	（ ）, product, deduce
	cleft, split	fiss-	fission
	fix, fasten	fix-	fixture, prefix
	flow	flu-	fluctuate, flux, fluid
	break	fract-	（ ）, refract
	stick to	here-, hes-	adhere, cohere, cohesion
	loose, break	lys-, lyz-	（ ）, lysemia
	mix	misc-, mix-	mixture, immiscible
	form, shape	morph-	metamorphosis, morphology
	love （fear）	phil- （phob-）	hydrophilic, （ ）
	full, maximize	sat-	saturated fatty acid, saturation binding
	dissolve	sol-	solution, water-soluble, solvent
	look	spec-	（ ）, special, spectrum
prefixes quality	sour, sharp	acid-, acri-, acu-	acute, （ ）, acrylic
	other, different	al-, allo-	alloy, alter, alias
	down, negative	cat-	cataphile, （ ）, catalyze
	cold	cry-	crystal, （ ）
	thick	dens-	density, condense
	basic	elem-	element, elementary school
	equal	equ-, iso-	（ ）, isotope, equilibrium
	sweet, sugar	glyc-	glycerol, （ ）, glycemia
	empty	vac-	vacuum, vacant, vacuous
suffixes	negatively charged ion	-ate, -ite	（ ）, nitrate, bromite
	single covalent bond	-ane	alkane, （ ）, ethane
	double covalent bond	-ene	alkene, ethylene, polyene
	triple covalent bond	-yne	alkyne, octyne
	higher valence	-ic	carbonic, ferric, acetic, sulfuric acid
	lower valence	-ous	sulfurous acid, nitrous, ferrous
	derived from	-ide	oxidative, bromide, （ ）
	describing	-ile	ductile, volatile, mobile
	unit	-on	（ ）, proton, boson

acidity	activity	catalysis	catalyst	conduct
crystalline	electron	equivalent	fraction	glycogen
hydrate	hydrophobic	methane	saccharide	spectator

9 B Look at a scientific text (e.g., scientific journals, textbooks, scientific news articles, etc.) and find 10 words that contain one (or more) affixes introduced in this unit. Write them in the box below.

word	affix	meaning	word	affix	meaning
1.			6.		
2.			7.		
3.			8.		
4.			9.		
5.			10.		

9 C Underline the affixes introduced in this unit and write the Japanese equivalent for each of the following terms.

1.   saturated   (   )
2.   equinox   (   )
3.   polysaccharide   (   )
4.   conduction   (   )
5.   acidophilic   (   )
6.   ethane   (   )
7.   caustic   (   )
8.   adhesion   (   )
9.   nuclear fission   (   )
10. catalysis   (   )

9 D Write the English equivalent for each of the following Japanese terms.

1.   電解質   (   )
2.   王 水   (   )
3.   グリセロール   (   )
4.   過飽和の（形）   (   )

Ⅳ   Scientific communication

10 Structure of a research article： The introduction

論文の構成Ⅰ： 序論（Introduction）

論文において，詳細な研究内容とその議論に相当するセクションをまとめて IMRaD（イムラド）とよびます．また，このような構成の論文を IMRaD 論文とよぶこともあります．IMRaD は，論文の構成セクションの序論（Introduction），方法（Methods），結果（Results），そして（and）考察（Discussion）のそれぞれの頭文字をとったものです．ここでは，序論（Introduction）はどのようなものかを見ていきましょう．

序論の構成

　文字通り，序論は本文の最初のセクションであり，読者が研究内容を理解するために必要な予備知識を提供するセクションです．序論には以下の構成要素が含まれます：背景，研究目的，仮説，研究方法，結果．本文の最初のセクションではありますが，多くの研究者はこのセクションを最後に執筆します．

背　景

　研究のテーマ・トピックの専門分野における位置づけを述べ，先行研究を引用しつつ，これまでどのようなことが明らかになっているか，および何が明らかになっていないのかを明確に示します．論旨の展開は，より一般的な内容からその研究のテーマ・トピックに焦点を絞るものになっています（general to specific）．

研究目的

　研究で明らかにしたいこと（リサーチクエスチョン），およびその重要性と意義が述べられています．研究目的には論理的根拠が必要です．主観的な意見ではなく，参考文献やデータなどを根拠に，その研究の目的を客観的に説明しています．

仮　説

　リサーチクエスチョンに関わる，研究によって具体的に検証可能な仮定を仮説といいます．仮説は，実験によって正しいことが検証できる（検証可能）か，正しくないことが検証できる（反証可能）必要があります．

研究方法

　仮説を検証するための方法の概略も序論には含まれます．研究方法がどのような点において先行研究とは異なるか，およびその意義も簡潔に記述します．

結　果

　研究目的が達成されたか否かを簡潔に記します．また，結果の重要性に関して言及することもあります．

11 Exercise

次の日本語に相当する英語を調べて書きなさい.

背　景 _____

目　的 _____

リサーチクエスチョン _____

論理的根拠 _____

仮　説 _____

検証可能（である）_____

反証可能（である）_____

Unit 5
Measurement and Instruments
We collected samples …

Unit 5 では以下の事柄を学びます.

I. Reading and listening

Topic 5　Sweetened Swimming Pools and Hot Tubs
"甘味料の入った水泳プール"の調査

1 Pre-reading activities

2 Reading text

3 Understanding the structure

4 Reading for details：Understanding methods of an experiment
実験の手順を理解する

5 Note-taking：Describing measurement and instruments
計測方法や計測機器について記述する

II. Language focus

6 Sentence patterns：Describing methods
研究方法を述べる・研究の材料，手順を示す

7 Application：Using the sentence patterns

III. Vocabulary and vocabulary learning skills

8 Words in the reading text

9 Word-formation：Affixes used in biomedical sciences
語形成：生物医科学系でよく使われる接辞を学ぶ

IV. Scientific communication

10 Structure of a research article：Methods and results
IMRaD 論文の構成：方法と結果について知る

11 Exercise

Workbook（Unit 5）▶ p. W 45

I   Reading and listening

Topic 5   Sweetened Swimming Pools and Hot Tubs

1   Pre-reading activities

1 A   Discuss the following with your partner.

1. Do you go to a public swimming pool?

2. When you go there, do you feel like you are swimming in a clean or unclean pool?

3. Why do you think you feel that way?

1 B   Listening activities   (Track 13)

1. Listen to the recording and write the keywords from the text.   ◀) **Track 13**

2. Listen again, paying attention to intonation, pronunciation, and pauses.

3. Read the text below aloud with the recording.

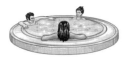

Hot tub

2   Reading text   (Track 13)

Topic 5

Sweetened Swimming Pools and Hot Tubs[9]

Abstract

Nitrogenous organics in urine can react with chlorine in swimming pools to form volatile and irritating N-Cl-amines. A urinary marker is desirable for the control of pool water quality. The widespread consumption of acesulfame-K (ACE), a stable synthetic sweetener, and its complete excretion in urine, makes it an ideal urinary marker. Here we report the occurrence of ACE and its potential application in swimming pools and hot tubs. First, we developed a new method for achieving high-throughput analysis of ACE without preconcentration or large-volume injection. Analysis of more than 250 samples from 31 pools and tubs from two Canadian cities showed ACE in all samples. Concentrations ranged from 30 to 7110 ng/L, up to 570-fold greater than in the input tap water. The level of dissolved organic carbon was significantly greater in all pools and tubs than in the input water. Finally, we determined the levels of ACE over 3 weeks in two pools (110,000 and 220,000 U.S. gallons) and used the average ACE level to estimate the urine contribution as 30 and 75 L. This study clearly shows the human impact in pools and tubs. This work is useful for future studies of the human contribution to DBP formation, epidemiological assessment of exposure, and adverse health effects in recreational facilities.

....

MATERIALS AND METHODS
Collection of Swimming Pool and Hot Tub Samples

We collected samples from two Canadian cities between May and August 2014. In city 1, samples were collected from 10 swimming pools (SP) and 5 hot tubs (HT) from 5 recreational facilities (RF) and 3 hotels (H). In city 2, samples were collected from 11 SPs and 3 HTs from 7 RFs and one private pool (P). All facilities used municipal tap water as the input source. Triplicate grab samples were collected using new, sterile, 15 mL polystyrene vials. In swimming pools and hot tubs, samples were collected away from the jets, approximately 30 cm from the edge and 15 cm below the surface. Municipal tap water was collected on the same day, in triplicate, at each site.

Samples were stored at 4 °C until they were analyzed. ACE is stable and resistant to decomposition, showing no detectable decrease in concentration after being stored for 10 years at room temperature. Samples were filtered through disposable 0.45 μm Millipore filters (PVDF, 25 mm). An analysis blank was injected into the HPLC-MS/MS instrument after each set of samples to detect and avoid any carryover or contamination during sequential analysis. No ACE was detected in the analysis blanks.

3   Understanding the structure

3 A   Text analysis

1. This reading includes the [   ] and [   ] of a research article.

2. Read the text once again and write the keywords from the text. Compare with the answers in "1 B Listening activities."

3. Choose one keyword from the above list and discuss it with your partner.

Your partner： What word did you choose？

You： I chose (   ).

Your partner： Can you explain the reason why you chose that word？

You： _____

3 B Skimming

1. What is the purpose of this study?

┌──┐
│   │
│   │
│   │
└──┘

2. Read the materials and methods section, and answer the following.

What is the purpose of the first paragraph？

┌──┐
│   │
│   │
│   │
└──┘

What is the purpose of the second paragraph？

┌──┐
│   │
│   │
│   │
└──┘

4 Reading for details： Understanding methods of an experiment

4 A Words in context

1. Find and circle the following verbs or their derived forms in the text. Choose one example sentence for each word from the reading and write it in the box.

develop

┌──┐
│   │
│   │
└──┘

collect

┌──┐
│   │
│   │
└──┘

determine

┌──┐
│   │
│   │
└──┘

analyze

store

filter

2. Find and underline the following materials.

> • new, sterile, 15 mL polystyrene vials　　• municipal tap water
>
> • disposable 0.45 μm Millipore filters （PVDF, 25 mm）

3. What was the purpose of using each material?

new, sterile, 15 mL polystyrene vials

municipal tap water

disposable 0.45 μm Millipore filters （PVDF, 25 mm）

4 B　Scanning: Where can you find the answers to the questions below? Underline the parts in the text. Discuss the answers with your partner.

1. Explain why the writer said swimming pools and hot tubs are sweetened in the title.

2. Explain why the writer thinks acesulfame-K is ideal as a urinary marker.

3. How many pools and tubs did they collect samples from?

4. Explain briefly how samples were stored?

4 C   Schematization and extension: Work in groups. Discuss the answers to the following questions.

1. Draw a picture that describes how a sample of water was collected from a hot tub.

2. How can we avoid contamination of swimming pools and hot tubs?
3. Are there other good markers to measure urine in swimming pools and hot tubs?

5   Note-taking: Describing measurement and instruments

Complete the chart below.

The objective	
Procedure 1	
Procedure 2	
Procedure 3	
Procedure 4	

Ⅱ   Language focus

6   Sentence patterns: Describing methods

In the methods section of a research article, the passive voice is typically used when the experimental procedure is described, whereas the active voice is preferred when the procedure is unique, or significant, in the study. Look at the following example:

> For mass spectrometry analysis, **samples** were **denatured, reduced,** and **alkylated** before an overnight digestion with trypsin.[10]

As the example suggests, the person who performed the actions is not mentioned. In scientific writing, the passive voice is used when it is not important to state the person who did the action.

In the methods section, the precise measurement of materials is given as well as the instruments used. In this unit, you will learn how to describe measurements and instruments.

Materials/instruments + was/were + a performing verb + (condition) .

Materials/instruments + was/were + a performing verb + purpose + (condition) .

Purpose + materials/instruments + was/were + a performing verb + (condition) .

1. materials/instrument: [   ]
2. a performing verb: _____
3. condition: (   )
4. purpose: to/for _____.

> [The membrane] <u>was then washed</u> (three times in PBST buffer) and <u>incubated</u> (with an anti-mouse HRP antibody).[11]

Performing verbs include: use, add to, incubate, mix with, obtain, perform, prepare, measure, stir, follow, wash, carry, record, collect, dissolve, remove, etc.

Inside the (condition) part comes the specific measurement and instrument.

Temperature: at _____ °C
Concentration: at _____ %, a concentration of _____ mM
Time: for _____ min, for _____ h
Frequency: _____ times
Instrument: using + a specific instrument, with + a specific instrument

Sentence patterns

1. [   ] **was** _____ (   ).
2. [   ] **was** _____ (   ) to ~~~~~~ .
3. [   ] **was** _____ (   ) that ~~~~~~ .
4. To/For ~~~~~~~~~~ [   ] **was** ~~~~~~~~~~~~ (   ).

Note: Many performing verbs take a specific preposition. It is important to learn the phrasal verbs frequently used in the methods section.

7   Application: Using the sentence patterns

Basic composition exercises

7 A   Paraphrasing: Look at the example sentences you wrote in "4 A Words in context." Rewrite each sentence in the boxes using sentence patterns introduced in this unit.

develop

collect

determine

analyze

store

filter

7 B Sentence completion: Fill in the blanks. Listen to the recording and check your answers.

1. The bacterial RNA genes in the DNA (   ) (   ) using the PCR technique and then sequenced (   ) high-capacity DNA sequencers.

2. The lungs of infected monkeys (   ) (   ) (   ) saline solution.

    ◀)) **Track 14**

3. (   ) document temperature and airflow speed, a vane anemometer (   ) (   ).

4. Calipers (   ) (   ) (   ) measure the skull structure.

7 C Oral exercise: Listen to the recording and answer the questions.

1. _____

2. _____

    ◀)) **Track 15**

3. _____

4. _____

Advanced composition exercises

7 D Work with your partner. Read the examples below and indicate each part of the method, using the notation system in the box.

> 1. materials/instruments: [   ]
> 2. a performing verb: _____
> 3. condition: (   )
> 4. purpose: to/for _____

Example: [**Samples**] were stored (at 4°C until they were analyzed).

1. In city 1, samples were collected from 10 swimming pools (SP) and 5 hot tubs (HT) from 5 recreational facilities (RF) and 3 hotels (H).

2. To modify NK cell function, mice were treated three times weekly either intravenously (i.v.) with an anti-Asialo-GM1 antibody (25 μl in 200 μl saline, Wako, USA) for 10 or 20 days or i.p. with poly I: C (Sigma, USA) 1 mg/kg.[12]

3. For *in vitro* cytotoxicity assays, growing or senescent cells were plated in 6-well plates at 50,000 cells per well.[13]

4. Concentrations of PFOS in liver and blood plasma were measured using high-performance liquid chromatography（HPLC）with electrospray tandem mass spectrometry.[14)]

7 E   Paraphrase each sentence in 7 D using your own words.

1. _____

   _____

2. _____

   _____

3. _____

   _____

4. _____

   _____

文型ノート: 受動態

　論文や論文要旨（**abstract**）において方法を説明する部分では受動態がよく使われ，一般の文章のように人の名前を主語にしたり，人称代名詞を主語にした文はあまり見られません．受動態は，他動詞の目的語を主語にして書く文のことですが，論文の作者が行った実験であれば，動作主が研究者本人であることが明確であるため，読者の注意を作者ではなく，実験動作そのものに向けるために受動態が用いられるのです．もしも実験の動作が特筆すべきものであるときには，**we** という複数の人称代名詞が使用されます．受動態の動詞の意味を知ると，**methods** 部分がやさしく感じられるようになります．

文法ノート: Use を使いこなそう！

　生命科学の分野を問わず **methods** 部分で圧倒的に多く用いられる動詞は **use** です．**Use** にはさまざまな用法があります．
1. 能動態の動詞 [〜を用いた] We used（使用したもの，分析方法，など）
2. 受動態の動詞 [〜が用いられた]（使用したもの，分析方法，など）was used as/to（用途／目的など）
3. 副詞的に [〜を用いて] using（使用したもの，分析方法，など）
4. 形容詞的に [〜で用いられた]（使用したもの，分析方法，など）used in（実験操作）

Ⅲ　　Vocabulary and vocabulary learning skills

8　Words in the reading text

8 A　Classify the words according to their parts of speech. There may be no words for a part of speech.

☐ adverse	☐ approximately	☐ assessment	☐ collect
☐ decomposition	☐ detect	☐ disposable	☐ epidemiological
☐ estimate	☐ excretion	☐ marker	☐ municipal
☐ nitrogenous	☐ occurrence	☐ range	☐ react
☐ resistant	☐ sample	☐ sequential	☐ source
☐ stable	☐ sterile	☐ tap water	☐ triplicate
☐ tub	☐ urine	☐ volatile	☐ volume

Check the box ☑ when you have learned the word.

nouns	verbs	adjectives	adverbs
assessment			

8 B　Choose four verbs from above and write a definition for each.

[　　　　　]　_____

[　　　　　]　_____

[　　　　　]　_____

[　　　　　]　_____

8 C　Discuss the terms above with your partner.

You：What does（　　　　）mean ?

Your partner：（　　　　）means _____.

9 Word-formation: Affixes used in biomedical sciences

Many words in biomedical sciences are derived from Greek and Latin words.

9 A Affixes often used in life sciences: Choose the words from the box on the next page to fill in the blanks.

function	meaning	affixes	examples
action	walk	ambul-	( ), amble, ambulance
	take	cep-, cept-	intercept, ( )
	to kill, to cut	cide-, cis-	( ), incision, germicide
	know, think	gno-	prognosis, diagnosis, ( )
	cut out	-ectomy	lumpectomy, ( )
	carry, bear	fer-	conifer, refer, infer
	bend	flex-, flect-	flexor, ( ), dorsiflex
	carry	gest-	gestation, congest, digest, ( )
	breathe	hal-, spir	halitosis, exhale, ( )
	join	junct-	conjunctive tissue, disjunction
	wander	migra-	migratory, migrate, ( )
	change	mut-, trop-	mutagen, ( ), tropomyosin, geotropism
	born, birth	nat-	innate, natal, ( ), postnatal
	smell	olfact-	( ), olfaction
	work	oper-	operation
	eat	phag-, vor-	macrophage, phagocyte, ( ), herbivorous
	carry	port-	( ), export, import
	know	sci-	science, conscious
	see, monitor	scop-, vid-, vis-	stethoscope, ( ), evident, revise
	write	script-	reverse transcriptase, ( )
	cut	sect-, tom-	( ), transect, microtome, anatomy
	feel	sens-	sensory, ( ), sensor
	save	serv-	conservationist, preserve
	touch	tact-, tag-	contagious, tactile, contact
	hold, stretch	ten-, tin-	tendon, retention, abstinent
quality	hidden	crypt-	( ), cryptozoa
	hard, lasting	dura-	( ), dura mater
	reddish	eryth-	erythrocyte, erythroblast
	safe	immun-	( ), immunology
	young	juven-	juvenile, rejuvenate

quality	soft	moll-	mollusk, emolliate, mollify
	mortal, death	mort-	postmortem, mortal
	new, recent	neo-	( ), neonate
	resemble, like	-oid	amoeboid, ( ), deltoid, thyroid
	straight, correct	ortho-	orthoptera, ( )
	seated, fixed	sed-, sess-	( ), sessile, residue
	alive, life	viv-, vita-	vitamin, vital, survive

ambulatory	appendectomy	cognitive	cryptic	dissect
durable	endoscope	esophagus	flexible	immigration
immunization	indigestion	mutant	native	neoplasm
olfactory	orthopedic	pesticide	portable	prescription
receptor	respiration	sedentary	sensation	steroid

9 B Look at a scientific text (e.g., scientific journals, textbooks, scientific news articles, etc.) and find 10 words that contain one (or more) affixes introduced in this unit. Write them in the box below.

	word	affix	meaning
1.			
2.			
3.			
4.			
5.			
6.			
7.			
8.			
9.			
10.			

9 C   Underline the affixes introduced in this unit and write the Japanese equivalent for each of the following terms.

1.   erythema   (   )
2.   phagocytosis   (   )
3.   omnivorous   (   )
4.   intact   (   )
5.   sensitize   (   )
6.   orthodontist   (   )
7.   autoimmunity   (   )
8.   juncture   (   )
9.   emigrate   (   )
10. adrenalectomy   (   )

9 D   Write the English equivalent for each of the following Japanese terms.

1.   自己貪食   (   )
2.   視 力   (   )
3.   消化不良   (   )
4.   予 後   (   )

Ⅳ   Scientific communication

10   Structure of a research article：Methods and results

論文の構成 Ⅱ：方法と結果

　序論において，研究方法と結果の概略は既に述べられていますが，方法と結果のセクションは，それぞれのより詳細な情報を提供するものです．それぞれどのような特徴があるか見ていきましょう．

方法（**Methods**）
　実際に行った研究手順と方法を記すセクションです．科学分野，学術学会／学術誌によっては，材料と方法，プロトコルなどとよぶこともあります．研究方法は，導き出された結果に信憑性があることを示し，論文を読んだ他の研究者が再現できる必要があります．そのために，次の内容を明確に記します：研究目的／計画，研究対象／材料，データ収集および分析方法．このセクションは，読者が研究結果や結論の妥当性を判断するための重要な情報提供であるため，明確さおよび正確さが求められます．

研究目的／計画
　　このセクションではより詳細な研究目的と研究計画を記述します．

研究対象／材料／手順
　　ここでは正確かつ具体的に，研究対象および研究に使用した材料や機器を記載します．

データ収集および分析方法
　　ここでは，研究計画に基づいて具体的な実験手順を書きます．どのようなデータをどのように収集するか，データ分析にはどのような方法を使用するか，分析の際に，除外する必要のあるデータがあれば，その除外基準が含まれます．

結果（**Results**）
　方法（Methods）のセクションに記載された方法で得られた結果を客観的に記すセクションです．つまり，このセクションでは，得られた結果に関する著者の見解などは一切記述しません．図表（Figure, Fig.；Table）を用いて主たる結果を示す場合が多く，それらの図表にはキャプション（caption：タイトルと短い説明）をつけます．本文でも必ずこれらの図表に言及します．

11 **Exercise**

次の日本語に相当する英語を調べて書きなさい.

プロトコル　　_____

信憑性　　　　_____

妥当性　　　　_____

研究対象　　　_____

研究材料　　　_____

データ収集　　_____

データ分析　　_____

表　　　　　　_____

グラフ　　　　_____

図　　　　　　_____

Unit 6
Results and Data Analysis
A paired *t*-test reveals …

Unit 6 では以下の事柄を学びます.

I. Reading and listening

Topic 6　Sweetened Swimming Pools and Hot Tubs
"甘味料の入った水泳プール"の分析結果

II. Language focus

III. Vocabulary and vocabulary learning skills

IV. Scientific communication

Workbook（Unit 6）▶ p. W 55

I   Reading and listening

Topic 6   Sweetened Swimming Pools and Hot Tubs

1   Pre-reading activities

1 A   Discuss the following with your partner.

1. Do you swim in a swimming pool or in the ocean? Which is cleaner?

2. Suppose some people, including small children, urinate in a public pool, what would be the best way to measure it?

3. What types of information do you expect to read in the results section?

4. What kinds of data do you expect to see in the study described in Unit 5?

1 B   Listening activities   (Track 16)

1. Listen to the recording and write five pieces of data you hear.

2. Listen again and compare your answers with your classmates.

3. Read the text below aloud with the recording.

2   Reading text   (Track 16)

◀)) Track 16

Topic 6

Sweetened Swimming Pools and Hot Tubs[9]

RESULTS AND DISCUSSION

Concentration of ACE in Swimming Pools and Hot Tubs

Figure 1 shows the concentrations of ACE determined in the pools and hot tubs. In city 1, the concentration of ACE in the pool samples ranged from 30 ng/L in SP10 to 2110 ng/L in SP8 (Figure 1a). In city 2, the concentration of ACE ranged from 90 to 580 ng/L in all the pools except SP20, where 1070 ng/L ACE was found (Figure 1b). ACE concentrations in all hot tub samples ranged from 70 to 100 ng/L (HT3, HT4, HT6, and HT7) and from 2220 to 7110 ng/L (HT1, HT2, HT5, and

HT8). HT5 contained the highest ACE concentration (7110 ng/L), more than double that of any other sample. These samples were collected at one time and represent only a snapshot in time. The large variation in the concentration of ACE in the pools and tubs may be explained by the water change cycling time point, the number of users and events, and facility management practices. Typically, fresh water is added to swimming pools only to maintain water levels, whereas hot tub water in community facilities is replaced frequently to prevent health issues associated with heavy use.

ACE was detected in all tap water samples at concentrations significantly lower than those in the pools and tubs in both cities. ACE in tap water samples ranged from 6 to 12 ng/L (Figure 2a) in city 1 and from 12 to 15 ng/L (Figure 2b) in city 2. The difference in ACE concentration in the two cities' tap waters is statistically significant ($p < 0.001$; unpaired t-test). This is expected, as the source water for each city is unique. The ACE concentrations in swimming pools and hot tubs were 4 (SP10) to 571 (HT5) times greater than that in the corresponding input tap water. The ACE concentrations determined in the tap water samples in this study are comparable to those of some Albertan well water samples (0.9–1530 ng/L ACE) and lower than those in Swiss tap waters (20–70 ng/L ACE).

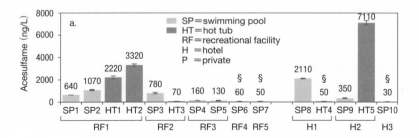

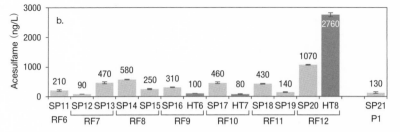

Figure 1. Average ACE concentration ($N=3$) detected in swimming pool (SP) and hot tub (HT) samples collected from public recreational facilities (RF), hotels (H), and a private residence (P) in (a) city 1 and (b) city 2. Samples indicated by the silcrow (§) were analyzed at a 1/10 dilution, rather than 1/20, because of their low ACE concentration.

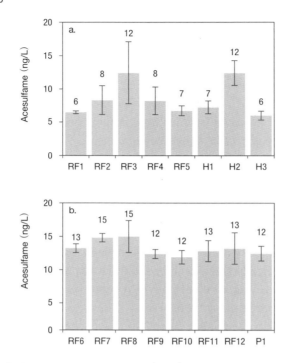

Figure 2. Average ACE concentration ($N=3$) detected in tap water samples collected from each sampling location in (a) city 1 and (b) city 2. The combined average of ACE concentration in each city's tap water was found to be statistically different using an unpaired Student's t-test ($p < 0.001$).

3 Understanding the structure

3 A Text analysis

1. How many samples were analyzed? There were [   ] samples in city 1 and [   ] samples in city 2.

2. What are the two sets of figures (Figure 1 and Figure 2) used in the text? What do they show?

Figure 1:
x- axis:
y- axis:
Figure 2:
x- axis:
y- axis:

3 B   Skimming

1. What does this text describe?

2. What does each paragraph describe?

4   **Reading for details: Understanding figures and interpretations**

4 A   Words in context

1. Underline the parts in the reading that show the following. Write the description for each in the boxes below.

ng/L

(   ) to (   )

the purpose of using a Student's *t*-test

2. What do the following abbreviations stand for? Write them out.

ng: _____   L: _____

ACE (Unit 5): _____

N: _____   HT: _____

4 B   Scanning: Where can you find the answers to the questions below? Discuss the answers with your partner.

1. Discuss the similarities and differences between Figure 1 and Figure 2.

2. Compare the concentration of ACE for the following pairs.

Ranges of ACE in swimming pools in city 1 and city 2

Ranges of ACE in hot tubs in city 1 and city 2

Ranges of ACE in tap water samples collected in city 1 and city 2

4 C   Comprehension : Discuss the answers to the following questions.

1. Where did the researchers find the highest concentration of ACE ?

2. Why do you think HTs generally contains more ACE than SPs ?

3. Based on what the authors claim, why do some HTs contain very small amounts of ACE ?

4. The authors report that the concentration of ACE in tap water is different in city 1 and city 2. Which city's tap water has a higher concentration of ACE ? Which evidence supports this claim ?

5   Reading graphs

Look at the graph and answer the following questions.

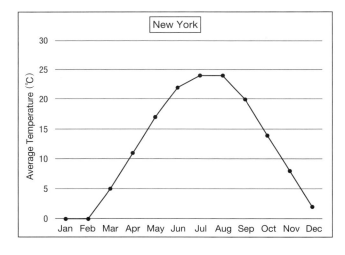

1. What graph is this ?

2. Which part of the graph is the *x*-axis ?

3. Which part of the graph is the *y*-axis ?

4. Write a brief description of what the graph shows. Be sure to describe the trend/s.

5. Write an appropriate title for the graph.

Figure _____

II	**Language focus**

6 Sentence patterns: Describing the results (figures, tables and numbers)

In the results section of research articles, the authors present the results they obtained through their study. The results section often contains a lot of figures, tables and numbers with specific notations. In addition, statistical analyses are given in the results section.

When you read the results, it is important to keep in mind what the numbers mean. In examples (1) to (3), the underlined part is what the author is describing, and the subsequent part is the results with figures. (4) and (5) show how tables and figures are explained.

(1) **[Description of simple measurement]**

In city 1, the **concentration** of ACE in the pool samples **ranged from** 30 ng/L in SP10 to 2110 ng/L in SP8.

Verbs include: was, were, ranged from (A to B)

(2) **[Results of measurement/analysis]**

The subject of the analysis	+	was/were	+	figures	.

Calcium sequestering activity of liver microsomes from control rats **was** 131.9 ± 10.1 nmol/mg protein per 60 min.[15)]

(3) **[Statistical analysis]**

The method of analysis	+	a verb	+	a statement of results	+	(figures)	.

The ANOVA **found** that model type had a significant impact on the percent reached [$F_{(2, 5398)} = 83.91$, $p < 0.001$].

A paired t-test **reveals** a significant difference between the two groups.

Verbs include: was, were, detected, shows/ed, found, reveals/ed, etc.

(4) **Referring to a table or chart**

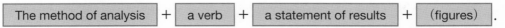

Table # / Figure #	+	a verb	+	a statement of results	.

Figure 1 shows the concentrations of ACE determined in the pools and hot tubs.

Verbs include: gives, demonstrates, displays, indicates, shows, compares, presents, provides, illustrates, summarizes, etc.

(5)   Interpretation of data (describing trends)

Types of graphs and charts

line graphs, bar graphs, pie charts, spider charts, scatter plots, histograms, Venn diagrams

Parts of graphs：

line, bar, part, portion, axis, horizontal line, the horizontal axis, the x-axis, vertical line, the vertical axis, the y-axis, legend, title, independent variable, dependent variable

Trends

nouns： an increase, a decrease, no change

adjectives： high, low, large, small, sharp, rapid, massive, considerable, huge, significant, insignificant, minimal

verbs： increase, rise, go up, grow, turn upward, reach a peak, reduce, decrease, dip, fall, drop, decline, plunge, go down, bottom out, reach a low, remain flat, remain constant, level off, stabilize, plateau, stagnate, stay flat, flatten out, remain still, keep pace, keep the same trend, fluctuate, zig-zag, flutter, undulate, occupy (ratio)

adverbs describing trends： significantly, substantially, markedly, moderately, somewhat, slightly, a little, roughly, above, below

adverbs describing the speed of change： quickly, rapidly, gradually, steadily, slowly, suddenly

intensifiers： as high as, as low as, to peak at, hit bottom at

Statistics

descriptive statistics： average, mean, median, mode, standard deviation, variance, kurtosis, skewness

parametric statistics： Student's t-test, Pearson correlation, analysis of variance (ANOVA)

nonparametric statistics： Chi-squared test (χ^2 test), Mann-Whitney U, Wilcoxon signed rank test

distribution： continuous distribution, normal distribution, discrete distribution

Sentence patterns

1. [measurement] <u>ranged from</u> (data) to (data).

2. [measurement] <u>was</u> (data).

3. [Statistical analysis] + <u>reveals</u> + that {   }

4. (table/figure) + <u>shows</u> + that {   }

7 **Application: Using the sentence patterns**

Basic composition exercises

7 A   Paraphrasing: Use the information from the reading and write a description of each of the following items. Use your own words.

ACE concentrations in city 1.

The highest concentration of ACE

ACE concentrations of tap water samples

Comparison between tap water samples in city 1 and city 2

7 B   Sentence completion: Fill in the blanks. Listen to the recording and check your answers.

1. The participants' ages (   ) (   ) 29 to 50.

2. The luminous intensity of the red LEDs (   ) about 50 (   ) 75 mcd (millicandela).

3. Cronbach's alpha (   ) (   ) only one strategy had low but acceptable internal consistency (alpha = 0.626).

4. Figure 1 (   ) the cumulative germination for *Capsicum annuum* seeds after the pre-germination treatment of soaking (   ) three days in a sodium chloride solution.

🔊 Track 17

7 C   Oral exercise: Listen to the recording and answer the questions. (1～4)

1. _____

2. _____

3. _____

🔊 Track 18

4. _____

Advanced composition exercises

7 D Work with your partner. Read the examples below and indicate each part of the description of the results, using the notation system in the box.

> 1. measurement / statistical analysis：[   ]
> 2. a verb to indicate the result：_____
> 3. data：《   》
> 4. table / figure：(   ).
> 5. results：{   }

1. Normal morning cortisol levels ranged from 10 to 20 micrograms per deciliter (mg/dL).

2. The temperature of the cooled liquid helium-4 was 1 K (kelvin).

3. Pearson's chi-squared tests showed the participants' responses for the association strategy were not statistically different for Group 1 and Group 2 at 0.5 level of significance (χ^2(1) $= 0.30$, $p = 0.78$ for association).

4. Table 2 provides the TOEIC scores of all the participants.

7 E Paraphrase each sentence in 7 D using your own words.

1. _____

_____

2. _____

_____

3. _____

_____

4. _____

_____

文型ノート：データの解釈

　論文において実験から得られたデータは，読者に伝えるためわかりやすく可視化する必要があります．グラフや図・写真は，Figure（Fig. / fig.）として通し番号をつけ，文中で適宜引用し，横や下に解説をつけて、その重要性を説明します．統計処理はグラフを用いて説明することが多く，数値も記載されています．研究論文を読むときに，abstract を読んだ後に，まず figure を見る研究者が多いのは，その論文に含まれる重要な発見は，必ずデータに示されているからです．データにはテクニカルな表現が多く含まれますが，論文を真に理解するには，示されたデータをクリティカルに（論理性，正確性，妥当性などを検討しながら）読むという作業が欠かせません．

文法ノート：単数と複数

　科学では，もともと不可算名詞（抽象名詞）だったものが可算名詞として使われていることがよくありますが，日本語には可算名詞，不可算名詞の区別がないので，気をつける必要があります．たとえば，Reading のテキストにある "concentration" は［濃度］という意味ですが，この単複は，文脈で使い分けます．

具体的な単位としての濃度

• a ＋ 単数形：濃度の単位を示すとき

"at a concentration of ＿ ng/L"　［1 L あたり＿ng の濃度］

• the ＋ 単数形：一つのサンプルの濃度を示すとき.

"the concentration of ACE in ~"　［～における ACE の濃度は］

• 複数形：複数のサンプルの濃度をまとめて示すとき.

"Figure 1 shows the concentrations of ACE…"　［Figure 1 は（それぞれのサンプルに含まれる）ACE の濃度を示している］

抽象的な意味の濃度

• 冠詞がつかない

"increase in concentration"　［濃度の増加］

濃度のような単位を表すものだけでなく，物質名詞も加算名詞で扱われるときがあります．これは個数ではなく量で表すもの（物質など）とそれらが複数の種類をもつときの意味の違いです．

例：tissue ＝組織

　　adipose tissue［脂肪組織］普通は不可算名詞

種類があることを示して使うとき（同種のものが複数あり，それらをまとめて言うとき）

　　brown and white adipose tissues　［褐色および白色脂肪組織］

物質の三態を表すときは可算名詞として使われることが多い.

　　Carbon dioxide is a gas at room temperature.　［二酸化炭素は室温で気体である.］

　　At temperatures below $-78\,^\circ\mathrm{C}$, carbon dioxide condenses into a solid.　［摂氏マイナス 78 度で二酸化炭素は固体に凝縮する.］

　　Liquid nitrogen is a colorless liquid.　［液体窒素は無色の液体である.］

| III | **Vocabulary and vocabulary learning skills** |

8 Words in the reading text

8 A Write the part of speech for each word in the parentheses. Use these abbreviations: noun = n; verb = v; adjective = adj; adverb = adv

Write the strategy you would use to learn these words in the brackets (see Study Guide pp. 5–8). You can use oral or writing rehearsal but try to use a deeper strategy. Combining more than two strategies is also effective (e.g., image and oral).

☐ average (n. adj.)	☐ contain ( )	☐ corresponding ( )	☐ determine ( )
[Association]	[ ]	[ ]	[ ]
☐ dilution ( )	☐ facility ( )	☐ figure ( )	☐ issue ( )
[ ]	[ ]	[ ]	[ ]
☐ maintain ( )	☐ replace ( )	☐ represent ( )	☐ residence ( )
[ ]	[ ]	[ ]	[ ]
☐ snapshot ( )	☐ statistically ( )	☐ table ( )	☐ typically ( )
[ ]	[ ]	[ ]	[ ]
☐ unique ( )	☐ variation ( )	☐ well water ( )	☐ whereas ( )
[ ]	[ ]	[ ]	[ ]

Check the box ☑ when you have learned the word.

8 B Discuss how you learned the terms above with your partner.

your partner: How did you learn ( ) ?

you: I used _____ to learn the word. Here's how I used the strategy. [You can show your partner how you used the strategy.]

8 C In order to succeed in learning a language, increasing vocabulary is key. Get in groups and share your opinions about which strategies you think are effective for RETAINING words. Did learning how to use deeper strategies affect your vocabulary learning? Write your conclusion after the discussion.

9   Word-formation: Frequently used roots in life sciences

9 A   Roots often used in life sciences: Listen to the recording and fill in the blanks.

🔊 Track 30

meaning	roots	examples
life	bio	( )
color	chromo	( )
cell	cyte, cyto	( )
water	hydro, hydor, aqua	aquarium
plant	herba	( )
egg	oo, ovum, ovi	oocyte
poison	tox, toxikon	( )
animal	zo, zoon	protozoa
child	pedi	( )
male	andro	( )
man	homo	( )
head	cephal, cephalon	cephalic
skin	derm, dermis	ectoderm
foot	pes, pedis, pod	( )
body	soma	somatic cell, lysosome
nerve	neuro	( )
feed, eat	trophe	( )
killing	cide	( )
marriage	gam, game	monogamy, gamete
origin	genesis, genic	( ), genotype
race, kind	genos, gen, geny	genealogy, genetics
disease, inflammation	itis	appendicitis, arthritis
destruction	lys, lysis	( ), hemolysis, hydrolysis
the study of	logos, logy	methodology, epidemiology
light	photo, phos, phot	( )

9 B Look at a scientific text (e.g., scientific journals, textbooks, scientific news articles, etc.) and find 10 words that contain a root introduced in this unit. Write them in the box below.

	word	root	meaning		word	root	meaning
1.				6.			
2.				7.			
3.				8.			
4.				9.			
5.				10.			

9 C Underline the roots introduced in this unit and write the Japanese equivalent for each of the following terms.

1. bioactivity   (   )
2. oocyte   (   )
3. encephalitis   (   )
4. pedestrian   (   )
5. somatic cells   (   )
6. zodiac signs   (   )
7. polygamy   (   )
8. herbicide   (   )
9. hydroelectric plant   (   )
10. pediatrist   (   )

9 D Write the English equivalent for each of the following Japanese terms.

1. 酔って（形）   (in   )
2. 動物学   (   )
3. 筋萎縮   (   )
4. 発電機   (   )

Ⅳ	**Scientific communication**

10 Structure of a research article： Discussion and references

論文の構成 Ⅲ： 考察と参考文献

　考察は論文において最も重要なセクションです．執筆の際には，最も難しくかつ最も時間を費やすセクションでもあります．論文では，研究において参考にした先行研究や執筆において引用をした先行研究およびその他文献を明示しなければなりません．参考文献は，本論を構築するセクションではありませんが，これがないものは論文とよぶことはできません．最後に，これら二つのセクションの目的と意義を見ていきましょう．

考察（Discussion）

　考察は，序論で述べた研究課題／テーマに対しての結論に至るまでの議論（discussion）に相当するセクションであり，ここでは，結果（Results）で示したデータに基づき，自身の主張を展開し，研究の結論および意義を示します．考察には次の内容が含まれます．

分析／主張

　　結果で示したデータを分析し，序論での問題提起（リサーチクエスチョン），仮説に対する研究の貢献（問題解決か否かなど）を主張します．

研究の意義

　　序論で示したリサーチクエスチョンに対する研究の学術的意義を述べます．

今後の発展／展望

　　当該研究分野での今後の研究の課題，方向性および将来性や，自身の研究をふまえての提言を述べます．

参考文献（References）

　1 つの研究は，それだけで成果が得られたものではなく，それまでに発表された研究の成果の上に発展させたものです．よって，先行研究に言及する場合は出典を示し，参考文献リストに掲載する必要があります．参考文献を明示することにより，次のことが達成されます．当該研究と先行研究の関連性が明確になること，科学的根拠のもとに実施された研究であること，先行研究に対する敬意の表明，読者への情報提供などです．参考文献はリストとして作成しますが，作成のフォーマットは学会やジャーナルによって異なるので，論文の投稿先がどのような投稿スタイルを採用しているか，投稿規定を確認し，作成する必要があります．

11 Exercise

Cell と *Nature* の参考文献リストを比べて気づいたことを箇条書きにしなさい.

> ・出版年の位置が *Cell* は著者の後だが *Nature* は一番最後である.

本書の二つの参考文献リスト（p.103 と p.W67）はそれぞれ違うジャーナルのスタイルを使用しています．それぞれどのジャーナルですか.

Textbook のスタイル [   ]   Workbook のスタイル [   ]

Textbook

References

1. Knols, B. G. J. On human odour, malaria mosquitoes, and Limburger cheese. *The Lancet* **348**, doi:10.1016/s0140-6736(05)65812-6 (1996).

2. Owino, E. A. Sampling of An.gambiae s.s mosquitoes using Limburger cheese, heat and moisture as baits in a homemade trap. *BMC Research Notes* **4**, 284, doi:10.1186/1756-0500-4-284 (2011).

3. Takahashi, K. & Yamanaka, S. Induction of pluripotent stem cells from mouse embryonic and adult fibroblast cultures by defined factors. *Cell* **126**, 663–676, doi:10.1016/j.cell.2006.07.024 (2006).

4. Bahl, V., Jacob, P., 3rd, Havel, C., Schick, S. F. & Talbot, P. Thirdhand cigarette smoke: factors affecting exposure and remediation. *PLoS ONE* **9**(10), e108258, doi:10.1371/journal.pone.0108258 (2014).

5. Haseleu, J., Omerbasic, D., Frenzel, H., Gross, M. & Lewin, G. R. Water-induced finger wrinkles do not affect touch acuity or dexterity in handling wet objects. *PLoS ONE* **9**(1), e84949, doi:10.1371/journal.pone.0084949 (2014).

6. Dai, A., Luo, D., Song, M. & Liu, J. Arctic amplification is caused by sea-ice loss under increasing CO_2. *Nature Communications* **10**, 121, doi:10.1038/s41467-018-07954-9 (2019).

7. Ramirez, A. *et al.* Hereditary parkinsonism with dementia is caused by mutations in ATP13A2, encoding a lysosomal type 5 P-type ATPase. *Nature Genetics* **38**, 1184–1191, doi:10.1038/ng1884 (2006).

8. Barateau, A. *et al.* Distinct Fiber Type Signature in Mouse Muscles Expressing a Mutant Lamin A Responsible for Congenital Muscular Dystrophy in a Patient. *Cells* **6**, doi:10.3390/cells6020010 (2017).

9. Jmaiff Blackstock, L. K., Wang, W., Vemula, S., Jaeger, B. T. & Li, X.-F. Sweetened Swimming Pools and Hot Tubs. *Environmental Science & Technology Letters* **4**, 149–153, doi:10.1021/acs.estlett.7b00043 (2017).

10. Papp, S. J. *et al.* DNA damage shifts circadian clock time via Hausp-dependent Cry1 stabilization. *eLife* **4**, doi:10.7554/eLife.04883 (2015).

11. Carrara, M., Prischi, F., Nowak, P. R., Kopp, M. C. & Ali, M. M. Noncanonical binding of BiP ATPase domain to Ire1 and Perk is dissociated by unfolded protein CH1 to initiate ER stress signaling. *eLife* **4**, doi:10.7554/eLife.03522 (2015).

12. Krizhanovsky, V. *et al.* Senescence of activated stellate cells limits liver fibrosis. *Cell* **134**, 657–667, doi:10.1016/j.cell.2008.06.049 (2008).

13. Chien, Y. *et al.* Control of the senescence-associated secretory phenotype by NF-kappaB promotes senescence and enhances chemosensitivity. *Genes & Development* **25**, 2125–2136, doi:10.1101/gad.17276711 (2011).

14. Kannan, K. *et al.* Accumulation of perfluorooctane sulfonate in marine mammals. *Environmental Science & Technology* **35**, 1593–1598, doi:10.1021/es001873w (2001).

15. Benedetti, A., Fulceri, R. & Comporti, M. Inhibition of calcium sequestration activity of liver microsomes by 4-hydroxyalkenals originating from the peroxidation of liver microsomal lipids. *Biochimica et Biophysica Acta (BBA) - Lipids and Lipid Metabolism* **793**, 489–493, doi:10.1016/0005-2760(84)90268-6 (1984).

Workbook

各 Unit とも以下の問題は音声を聞いて答える問題です．教員
の指示に従って下さい．
  1. Reading B
  2. Language focus C,D（ただし，Unit 6 にはありません）
  3. Vocabulary D（Unit 6 は C）

Unit 1　1. Reading

check

Class _____　I.D. _____　Name _____

A. Read the text and mark T if the statement is true. Mark F if the statement is false and rewrite the sentence.

1. (T　F)　In the first paragraph, there are four diseases that are given as examples of diseases transmitted by mosquitoes.

_____

2. (T　F)　Mosquitoes are more attracted to human males than females.

_____

3. (T　F)　We attract more mosquitoes after eating certain foods.

_____

4. (T　F)　As we exercise, we increase the amount of lactic acid in our body.

_____

5. (T　F)　The name of the bacteria found between our toes tells you that the bacteria have something to do with skin.

_____

6. (T　F)　Limburger cheese is fermented with *B. epidermidis*.

_____

7. (T　F)　The results of the gas chromatographic analyses showed that the chemical composition of a substance in the odor of Limburger cheese and in toe-nail scrapings are alike.

_____

8. (T　F)　*Anopheles gambiae* is the name of a microorganism commonly found in Limburger cheese and toe-nail scrapings.

_____

9. (T　F)　One researcher in Africa is trying to capture mosquitoes that may transmit malaria by using a cheese trap.

_____

B. Listen to the recording and write the answers below.

1.

2.

3.

C. Write the thesis statement and the main idea of each of the body paragraphs.

The thesis statement of the text:

_____

Paragraph 1:

_____

Paragraph 2:

_____

Paragraph 3:

_____

Paragraph 4:

_____

Paragraph 5:

_____

Unit 1 **2. Language focus**

Class _____ I.D. _____ Name _____ check

A. Read the sentences below and indicate each part of the definition, using the notation system in the box below.

> 1. the word to be defined： [   ]
> 2. a defining verb： ~~~~~~~~~~
> 3. the general class the word belongs to： (   )
> 4. specific characteristics： _____

1. Ecology refers to the study of natural systems, emphasizing the interdependence of one element in a system on every other element.　(Lawton and Nahemow, 1973: 619)

2. Intestinal failure (IF) was first defined in 1981 by Fleming and Remington as "a reduction in the functioning gut mass below the minimal amount necessary for adequate digestion and absorption of food."　(Pironi *et al.*, 2015: 172)

3. The metabolic syndrome can be defined as a state of metabolic dysregulation characterized by insulin resistance, central obesity, and a predisposition to type 2 diabetes, dyslipidemia, premature atherosclerosis, and other diseases.
　　　　　　　　　　　　　　　　　　　　(Ruderman and Saha, 2006: 25S)

4. Induced pluripotent stem cells (iPSCs) are adult cells that have been genetically reprogrammed to an embryonic stem cell-like stage by being forced to express genes and factors important for maintaining the defining properties of embryonic stem cells.　(Ghaedi *et al.*, 2015: 82)

5. By definition, **alkenes** are hydrocarbons with one or more carbon-carbon double bonds $(R_2C=CR_2)$, while **alkynes** are hydrocarbons with one or more carbon-carbon triple bonds $(R-C\equiv C-R)$. Collectively, they are called **unsaturated hydrocarbons**, which are defined as hydrocarbons having one or more multiple (double or triple) bonds between carbon atoms.　(Abozenadah *et al.*, 2017: 4)

B. Paraphrase each sentence above using your own words. (1～5)

1. _____

_____

2. _____

_____

3. _____

_____

4. _____

_____

5. _____

_____

C. Fill in the blanks. Listen to the recording and check your answers.

1. Moh's scale (   ) (   ) (   ) for (   ) minerals
   based on relative hardness, determined (   ) the ability of harder minerals to
   scratch (   ) ones.

2. Bituminous coal (   ) (   ) relatively soft (   ) containing a
   tarlike substance called bitumen or asphalt.

3. An emoji (   ) (   ) small icon that (   ) be placed inline
   with text.

4. Quartz refers (   ) (   ) family of crystalline gemstones of various
   colours and sizes.

5. Irrigation may (   ) defined (   ) the science of artificial application
   of (   ) to the land or soil.

D. Dictation: Listen to the recording and write what you hear.

1. _____

2. _____

Unit 1　3. Vocabulary

Class _____　I.D. _____　Name _____　[check]

A.　Choose appropriate words/phrases from the box below to
　　complete the sentences.

1.　We (　　　　　) that the reason why Limburger cheese and feet have a similar
　　(　　　　　) is that they have some (　　　　　) from the same genus. We
　　conducted an experiment to find (　　　　　) for the hypothesis.

2.　The cheese is made in a (　　　　　) environment (　　　　　) to that of
　　human feet.

3.　Insects that (　　　　　) on blood can act as (　　　　　) and (　　　　　)
　　diseases from person to person.

4.　Many diseases including cancer are (　　　　　) with smoking.

5.　Humans inhale oxygen and (　　　　　) carbon dioxide.

6.　Scientists are trying to create (　　　　　) versions of carboxylic fatty
　　(　　　　　).

7.　The trap (　　　　　) our knowledge of mosquito behavior to attract them.

8.　A parasite lives in a (　　　　　), which is usually a larger (　　　　　).

acids	associated	comparable	evidence
exhale	harnesses	host	hypothesized
microorganisms	moist	odor	organism
subsist	synthetic	transmit	vectors

B. Define the following words using the sentence patterns in this unit. Make sure you use a different sentence pattern for each.

1. octopus: _____

2. kilogram: _____

3. triangle: _____

4. centipede: _____

5. microwave oven: _____

C. What are these? Write the words or phrases below.

1. (   )

1.

2. adenosine (   )

3. km = (   )

2.

4. 128 GB = 128 (   )

5. ng = (   )

D. Dictation: Listen to the recording and write the words or sentences you hear.

1. _____

2. _____

3. _____

4. _____

5. _____

Unit 1   4. Reading glossary

a variety of	種々の
acid	酸
Anopheles gambiae	ハマダラカ
appeal	魅力を訴える，アピールする
associate（with）	関わる，関連する（be associated with）
attract	ひきつける，魅惑する，誘引する
bacteria	細菌，バクテリア
bait	餌
bite	咬傷，刺す
blend	混合，混合物，混ぜる
body region	身体領域，体部位
borne	（接尾辞的に）媒介性の
Brevibacterium	（グラム陽性菌の一属）ブレビバクテリウム，ブレビバクテリウム
carbon dioxide	二酸化炭素，炭酸ガス
carboxylic	カルボキシの
chemical	化学の，化学的な，化学物質，化学薬品，ケミカル
comparable	類似の，同等の，比較できる
confirm	確認する，確信させる，確証させる，確かめる
coryneform	（微生物分類）コリネ型の
deadly	致命的な，命にかかわる
dengue fever	（蚊が媒介するウイルス感染症）デング熱
distinctive	特有の，特徴的な
due to	…が原因で，…のために，…のせいで
evidence	証拠，根拠，証明
exhale	息を吐き出す，呼息する
factor	因子，要因，要素，ファクター
fatty acid composition	脂肪酸組成
feed	（餌を）与える，摂食する
genus	（分類学）属
harness	利用する
hematophagous	吸血性の
host	宿主，供給者
hypothesize	仮定する
insect	昆虫
itchy	痒い
Japanese encephalitis	日本脳炎
lactic acid	乳酸
malaria	マラリア

Track 19

microorganism	微生物
moist	湿性の
moisture	水分，湿気
mosquito	蚊
mosquito bite	蚊咬傷
noticeable	目につきやすい
notion	考え，意見，概念，観念
odor	匂い，臭気
organism	生物，生命体，生物体
possibility	可能性
potential	可能な，有望な，潜在的な，能力，可能性
pregnant woman	妊婦
pungent	刺激的な，鼻につんとくる
remarkably	著しく，目立って，際だって
responsible	原因となる，責任がある
scale	規模
scraping	剥離物
sense of smell	嗅覚
sensu stricto	（学名に後置するラテン語形容詞）厳密な意味での
species	種，菌種，種属
stand out	目立つ，優れる
sweat	汗
synthetic	合成された，合成の，合成的な
thrive	栄える
toe	足指，趾，つま先
toenail	趾爪，足指爪
track	追跡する
transmission	病気の伝播，感染，伝染
transmit	伝達する，透過する，伝える，伝染させる
trap	捕まえる，捉える，閉じ込める
vector	媒介動物，媒介者
vigorously	活発に，勢いよく
virus	ウイルス（生物と非生物のあいだに位置する微小構造体）

Unit 1　5. Word-formation samples

biannual	年2回の	nullisomy	零染色体性
binary	二進法の	octagon	八角形
centimeter	センチメートル	octamer	八量体
centipede	ムカデ	octane	オクタン
decade	10年間	octanol	オクタノール
decamer	十量体	octopus	タコ
decane	デカン	oligophagous	少食性
decapoda	十脚類	paucity	少数
December	12月	pentagon	五角形
decimal	十進法の	picogram	ピコグラム
decimal point	小数点	polyphenol	ポリフェノール
dichotomy	二分割	primitive	原始の
duodenum	十二指腸	protozoa	原生動物
duplicate	複製する	quadruple	4倍の
dyad	二分染色体	quarterly	年4回の
gigabyte	ギガバイト	quintan fever	五日熱
hectopascal	ヘクトパスカル	quintet	5人組
hemisphere	半球，脳半球	quintuple	5倍の
heptad	七つ組の	quintuplet	五つ子
heptagon	七角形	secondary	二次的な
heptamer	七量体	seminar	セミナー
hexagon	六角形	September	9月
kilogram	キログラム	sextuple	6倍の
megahertz	メガヘルツ	terabyte	テラバイト
megawatt	メガワット	tertiary	三次的な
micrometer	マイクロメートル	tetrapod	四肢動物
microwave oven	電子レンジ	tetragon	四角形
millimeter	ミリメートル	tetrakisphosphate	四リン酸
monosaccharide	単糖	total	総計の
multiplication	掛け算	totality	完全性
nanogram	ナノグラム	totipotency	全能性
nonamer	九量体	triangle	三角形
nonane	ノナン	triphosphate	三リン酸
November	11月	triplicate	3倍する
nullify	無効にする	trisomy	三染色体性
nullipotent	無能	unicellular	単細胞

Track 20

Unit

1

Unit 2   1. Reading

Class _____   I.D. _____   Name _____

A. Read the text and mark T if the statement is true. Mark F if the statement is false
    and rewrite the sentence.

1. (T F) PCR makes it possible for researchers to change DNA sequences.

_____

2. (T F) The DNA method is not only used in many fields of biology and medicine, but
           also in the field of history.

_____

3. (T F) The Russian Imperial Romanov family was arrested after the Russian
           Revolution.

_____

4. (T F) Two members of the Romanov family survived the revolution and lived until
           2007.

_____

5. (T F) Investigations using PCR revealed that Ötzi had died of an infectious disease.

_____

6. (T F) Eighteen living people have been identified as being genetically related to
           Ötzi.

_____

7. (T F) King Tut was 19 years old when he died.

_____

8. (T F) PCR was used to identify the remains of an English king.

_____

9. (T F) PCR is the only method used in the investigation of human remains.

_____

B. Listen to the recording and write the answers below.

1.

2.

3.

C. Write the thesis statement and the main idea of each of the body paragraphs.

The thesis statement of the text：

_____

Paragraph 2：

_____

Paragraph 3：

_____

Paragraph 4：

_____

✂

Unit 2   2. Language focus

Class _____   I.D. _____   Name _____   check

A. Read the sentences below and indicate each part of the classification or exemplification, using the notation systems in the boxes below.

Classification:

> 1. the concept to be classified: (   )
> 2. a classification verb: ＿＿＿＿＿
> 3. subdivisions: [   ]
> 4. classification number: ＿＿＿＿＿
> 5. classification nouns: 〈   〉

1. Beeswax can be classified generally into European and Oriental types.

2. There are two broad categories of fish: freshwater fish and marine fish.

3. There are mainly eight classifications of diseases: topographic, anatomic, physiological, pathological, etiologic (causal), juristic, epidemiological, and statistical.

Exemplification:

> 1. statement of concept or concept/noun phrase to be exemplified: [   ]
> 2. linking phrase: ＿＿＿＿＿
> 3. examples: (   )
> 4. exemplifying phrase: ＿＿＿＿＿

4. Some of the most common probiotics include *Bifidobacterium*, *Lactobacillus* and *Saccharomyces boulardii*, which is a type of yeast.

5. Several genes that are frequently upregulated in tumors, such as *Stat3*, *E-Ras*, *c-myc*, *Klf4*, and *β-catenin*, have been shown to contribute to the long-term maintenance of the ES cells in culture.   (Takahashi and Yamanaka, 2006: 663)

6. Nonetheless, it is clear that protein synthesis differs among mammalian somatic cells. For instance, cells of the exocrine pancreas display some of the highest rates of protein synthesis of any adult cell type.   (Buszczak *et al.*, 2014: 242)

B. Paraphrase two of the sentences above using your own words.

1. _____

_____

2. _____

_____

C. Fill in the blanks. Listen to the recording and check your answers.

1. Hematophagy can be (   ) (   ) obligatory and optional practice.

2. Vaccines that are currently available can be (   ) (   ) (   ) types: live virus vaccines that use the weakened form of the virus, killed vaccines that are made from a protein or other small pieces taken from a virus or bacteria, toxoid vaccines that contain a toxin or chemical made by the bacteria or virus, and biosynthetic vaccines that contain manmade substances similar to pieces of the virus or bacteria.

3. *Eschericia coli* can cause bacterial infections (   ) cholecystitis, bactermia, cholangitis, urinary tract infection, and other clinical infections.

4. Plant hormones are used in agriculture to have a specific effect. (   ) (   ), auxins are used as weed killers and rooting powders that promote growth, and gibberellins are used to end seed dormancy, promote flowering and increase fruit size.

5. These studies suggest that (   ) are four (   ) of fatigue in multiple sclerosis: (1) normal fatigue; (2) episodic fatigue; (3) continuous fatigue; and (4) myasthenic-like fatigue.

D. Dictation: Listen to the recording and write what you hear.

1. _____

2. _____

✂

Unit 2 3. Vocabulary

Class _____ I.D. _____ Name _____

check

A. Choose appropriate words/phrases from the box below to complete the sentences.

1. X-rays of King Tut's (   ) (   ) that he was about 19 years old when he died.

2. After the (   ) of the dynasty, the members of the (   ) family were all (   ), leaving no survivors.

3. Mary has a calm, relaxed (   ) which makes her popular with her friends.

4. We need to decide which (   ) to use to (   ) the mystery.

5. A DNA (   ) may be useful in (   ) who you are.

6. Last summer, we went on a hike to a (   ) in Yellowstone National Park. It was cold.

7. Scientific techniques such as (   ) have (   ) to our understanding of history.

8. DNA test kits can provide (   ) proof of our (   ).

carbon dating	collapse	conclusive	contributed
executed	glacier	identifying	imperial
kinship	method	mummy	revealed
segment	temperament	unravel	

B. Write either a classification sentence, an exemplification sentence, or a combination of the two with the following words using the sentence patterns in this unit. Make sure you use a different sentence pattern for each. (1〜4)

1. blood cells, red blood cells, white blood cells, platelets:

_____

2. soft drinks, carbonated (e.g., cola, ginger ale), noncarbonated (e.g., orange juice, tea):

_____

3. tetrapods, amphibians, reptiles, birds, mammals:

_____

4. infectious diseases, modes of transmission, direct contact (e.g., AIDS, hepatitis B), indirect contact (e.g., malaria, dengue fever):

_____

_____

_____

C. Underline the affixes in the following words, and then write the meaning of the affixes and the words.

Example: <u>annual</u> affix: [year] meaning: [covering the period of a year; occurring or happening every year or once a year]

1. chronic   affix: [   ] meaning: [   ]

2. microorganism affix: [   ] meaning: [   ]

3. distillation   affix: [   ] meaning: [   ]

4. interaction   affix: [   ] meaning: [   ]

5. endosome   affix: [   ] meaning: [   ]

D. Dictation: Listen to the recording and write the words or sentences you hear.

1. _____

2. _____

3. _____

4. _____

5. _____

Unit 2 4. Reading glossary

🔊 Track 21

amplify	増幅する
analyze	分析する，解析する
ancestor	祖先，先祖
ancient	古代の
application	適用，応用
armed force	軍隊
arrow	矢印，矢
blueprint	青写真
bone disease	骨疾患，骨系統疾患，骨障害
burial	埋葬，埋没
carbon dating	放射性炭素年代測定法
categorize	分類する，大別する，カテゴリー化する
characteristic	特徴的な，特有の，独特の，特徴，特性
collapse	崩壊
conclusively	決定的に，確証的に，結論的に
conduct	行う，遂行する
contribute	寄与する，貢献する，寄付する
declare	宣言する，公表する，明言する，断言する
determine	決定する，特定する，確定する，判定する，測定する，定量する
discovery	発見
DNA analysis	DNA 分析
evolve	進化する，発展する，発達させる
execute	実行する，遂行する，果たす，行う
gene	遺伝子
genetic	遺伝的な，遺伝子の，遺伝学的な，遺伝子的な，ジェネティックな
genetically	遺伝的に，遺伝学的に
glacier	氷河
high fidelity	ハイフィデリティー（忠実性が高い）
identification	同定，識別，個体識別
identify	（物や機能を）明らかにする，同定する，特定する，同一視する，確認する
indicate	指し示す，示す，意味する，指示する，表示する
intact	無傷の，そのままの状態の
investigate	研究する，精査する，検討する，調べる，調査する
investigation	研究，調査，検討，究明，（臨床）治験
kinship	血縁
linked	連鎖の，連鎖的な，連鎖性の
medicine	医学，薬
missing	あるべきところにない，行方不明の

multiple	複数の
mummy	ミイラ
organism	生物，生命体，生物体
PCR	
polymerase chain reaction	ポリメラーゼ連鎖反応法，核酸増幅法
positive	陽性の，正の，積極的な
possession	所有，所有物
preserve	保存する，貯蔵する，保つ
prisoner	囚人
procedure	手順，手続き，手技，術式，方法，製法，進め方，（法律）訴訟
remain	残る，残存する，…のままである，遺物，遺体，遺骨
remaining	残っている，残りの
reveal	明らかにする，暴露する，暴く
revolution	革命，大変革
risk	リスク，危険，危険性，危険度
segment	セグメント，区域，分節，体節，片
sequence	配列，連続，シークエンス
solve	（問題を）解決する，解く
Soviet Union	ソビエト連邦
specialty	専門，専門性，専門領域
specific	特定の，特異性の
standard	標準，標準的な
survivor	生存者
temperament	気質，気性
test tube	試験管
unravel	解決する，解明する
unsolved	未解決の，未解明の
X-ray	X線，エックス線
X-ray examination	X線検査

Unit 2　5. Word-formation samples

Track 22

aberration	異常
ablation	除去
adduct	付加物，内転させる
adhere	付着する
adjacent	隣接した
Alphaproteobacteria	アルファプロテオバクテリア
altimeter	高度計
altitude	高度
anhydrous	無水の
annual	一年の
antemortem	死ぬ前の
anterior	前方の
aquarium	水族館
biennial	2 年に 1 度の
centrifuge	遠心分離機
chronic	慢性の
chronoamperometry	クロノアンペロメトリー
coefficient	係数
compose	構成する
covalent	共有結合の
degrade	退化させる
diagonal	対角線の
diameter	直径
diffuse	放散する
disperse	分散させる
dissociate	分離する
distillation	蒸留
ectodomain	外部ドメイン
effluent	流出する
endogenous	内在性の
endosome	エンドソーム
epidemic	流行性の
epidermis	表皮
exoskeleton	外骨格
extract	抽出する
hemisphere	半球体
hyperbolic	双曲線の
hyperhydration	水分過剰
hypoxia	低酸素
infrared	赤外線の
interaction	相互作用
intracellular	細胞内の
locate	置く
locus	遺伝子座
macromonomer	マクロモノマー
macrophage	マクロファージ
medium	媒介物，媒体，培地
mesophilic	中温性の
microorganism	微生物
microscope	顕微鏡
nucleotide	ヌクレオチド
nucleus	細胞核
oligonucleotide	オリゴヌクレオチド
oligosaccharide	オリゴ糖
parallel	平行の，並行する
parameter	パラメーター
posterior	後部の
postmortem	死後の，検死
postnatal	出生後の
previously	以前に
primate	霊長目の動物
primer	プライマー
proceed	続行する
reaction	反応
reactor	化学反応器
reagent	試薬
semiconductor	半導体
substrate	基質
transfer	移す
ultrapure	超高純度の
ultrasound	超音波
ultraviolet	紫外線の

Unit 3   1. Reading

check

Class _____   I.D. _____   Name _____

A. Read the text and mark T if the statement is true. Mark F if the statement is false and rewrite the sentence.

Abstract 1

1. (T F)   Previous studies have revealed how to reduce THS components in fabrics.

_____

2. (T F)   TSNAs refer to chemical substances contained in THS.

_____

3. (T F)   Two kinds of fabrics were first exposed to smoke for 19 months.

_____

4. (T F)   The study revealed fleece can retain more toxic substances than cotton does.

_____

5. (T F)   The study concludes that THS is potentially more harmful more dangerous than secondhand smoke for both toddlers and adults.

_____

6. (T F)   Possible applications of the findings are not suggested in the abstract.

_____

Abstract 2

7. (T F)   The authors hypothesized that it might become easier to handle wet objects with wrinkled fingers.

_____

8. (T F)   There were 40 participants in the study.

_____

9. (T F)   This study proved water-induced skin wrinkling improves handling of wet objects.

_____

B. Listen to the recording and write the answers below.

1.

2.

3.

C. Take notes on each abstract.

Abstract 1

Background	
Objectives	
Materials	
Methods	
Major findings	
Conclusion	

Abstract 2

Background	
Objectives	
Participants	
Methods	
Major findings	
Conclusion	

Unit 3 | 2. **Language focus**

check

Class _____ I.D. _____ Name _____

A. Read the sentences below and indicate each part of the causal relationship, using the notation system in the box below.

---

1. [   ] : cause
2. ~~~~~~~~~~ : phrase to indicate causal relationship
3. (   ) : result

---

1. Second, nephrin must be crucial for the structural integrity of the slit diaphragm, as absence of the protein or different amino acid substitutions cause congenital nephrosis and lack of the slit diaphragm with massive proteinuria as a result.
   (Ruotsalainen *et al.*, 1999: 7965)

2. ELISA is less sensitive than the ELISPOT assay, and for this reason, we had to use a higher number of cells/mL in ELISA compared to ELISPOT.   (Hagen *et al.*, 2015: 87)

3. To investigate the ability of wearables to predict and monitor disease, a normalization framework was developed to accommodate the dynamic change caused by different activities and make measurements comparable.   (Li *et al.*, 2017: 2)

4. Although purified proteins were eluted in buffer with no added zinc, we cannot exclude the possibility that the purified proteins contributed some nonradioactive zinc to the reaction mixture.   (Warnhoff *et al.*, 2017: 21)

B. Paraphrase each sentence above using one of the sentence patterns introduced in this unit. (1～4)

1. _____

   _____

2. _____

   _____

3. _____

_____

4. _____

_____

C. Fill in the blanks. Listen to the recording and check your answers.

1. In mountainous areas very heavy rains often (   ) (   ) landslides.

2. Recent interest in rainwater harvesting (   ) (   ) (   ) drought and environmental awareness.

3. Earth's magnetic field is (   ) (   ) the flow of molten iron in the core.

4. The force of the earthquake was extremely strong. (   ) (   ) (   ), the earth's axis shifted 25 cms.

5. Human iPS cells (   ) (   ) (   ) (   ) every type of cell in the body.

6. The sand dunes (   ) (   ) by winds.

D. Dictation: Listen to the recording and write what you hear.

1. _____

2. _____

Unit **3** Vocabulary

Unit 3   3. Vocabulary

check

Class _____   I.D. _____   Name _____

A. Choose appropriate words/phrases from the box below to complete the sentences.

1. The palms and (   ) are sensory organs. They can recognize (   ) senses.

2. In order to be a good researcher, we need visual (   ) in making observations and (   ) in handling instruments.

3. Fabrics (   ) with tobacco smoke retained a (   ) amount of the (   ) of TSNAs after 19 months.

4. The researchers hypothesized that (   ) on fingers may have an (   ) on the handling of wet objects.

5. The (   ) of nicotine and other chemical (   ) in THS was investigated.

6. (   ) to forest fire smoke irritates our eyes, throat and nose, and we can develop lung and heart problems if we (   ) it.

7. (   ) tissue covers the outside of plants.

acuity	components	concentration	contaminated
dermal	dexterity	exposure	impact
inhale	residue	significant	soles
tactile	wrinkling		

B. Write sentences with the following words using the sentence patterns in this unit. Make sure you use a different sentence pattern for each.

1. deforestation： _____

2. malaria： _____

3. antigen： _____

4. vertebrates： _____

5. (your own)： _____

C. Write the opposite term for each of the following.

1. benevolent ←→ ( )

2. exoskeleton ←→ ( )

3. homogeneous ←→ ( )

4. internet ←→ ( )

5. utopia (eutopia) ←→ ( )

D. Dictation： Listen to the recording and write the words or sentences you hear.

1. _____

2. _____

3. _____

4. _____

Unit 3   4. Reading glossary

Track 23

abstract	要約，抄録，アブストラクト
acuity	鋭さ，鋭敏さ
aged	時間の経過した，高齢の
aging	時間効果，加齢，熟成
alkaloid	アルカロイド
aqueous	水性の，水の，水溶性の
chemical analysis	化学分析
cloth	布，布地
cohort	コホート，統計因子を共有する集団
component	成分，構成成分，構成要素
concentration	濃度，濃縮，集中
contaminate	混入する，汚染する
cotton	綿
dependent	依存性の，依存的な
dermal	皮膚の，経皮の，真皮の
dexterity	器用さ
estimate	推定，概算，見積，見積もる，推定する
evaluate	評価する，調べる
expose	曝露する，露出する，露光する，被曝する，曝す
exposure	曝露，被曝
extract	抽出する，抽出物
extraction	抽出，抽出法
fabric	織物，布
frame	骨組み，枠，フレーム
glabrous	無毛の
gross	全体の，総量の
hairy	毛様，毛髪状の，有毛の
handling	手を使ってものを扱うこと，取扱い
impact	衝撃，影響，インパクト，影響する
indoor	屋内の
induce	誘発する，誘起する，ひき起こす
infant	乳児
inhale	吸入する，吸引する
investigate	研究する，精査する，検討する，調べる，調査する
laboratory	研究室，実験室，検査室，ラボ
liquid chromatography	液体クロマトグラフィー
manual	手動の
measure	計測する，測る，方法，施策，処置，尺度，基準

nicotine	ニコチン
nitrosamine	ニトロソアミン
oral	経口の，経口的な
palm	手掌，手のひら
passive	受動的な，受動性の，受動の，消極的な
persist	持続する，存続する
physiology	生理学，生理，生理機能
polyester	ポリエステル
prolonged	長期間の，遷延性の，遷延した
public health	公衆衛生，公衆衛生学
remediation	治療
residue	残留物，残渣，残分，残基
retain	保持する，保定する
secondhand smoke	副流煙
sensation	感覚，感覚機能
sensitivity	感受性，感度，感応性，敏感性
sensory	感覚性の，感覚の，知覚性の
significant	統計的に有意な，意味ある，重要な，著しい
significant amount	相当量
skin wrinkling	皮膚のしわ
smoker	喫煙者
sole	足の裏，唯一の，単独の
strategy	戦略，計画，方略，ストラテジー
sympathetic nervous system	交感神経系
tactile	触覚の
tandem mass spectrometry	タンデム質量分析（法）
tobacco	タバコ
toddler	幼児
wrinkle	しわ，しわになる
wrinkling	しわ

Unit 3　5. Word-formation samples

amorphous	無定形の	ignore	無視する
anaerobic	嫌気的な	infrared	赤外線の
anomalous	変則の	innocuous	無害の
antibody	抗体	insane	狂気の
antigen	抗原	intercellular	細胞間の
antiseptic	防腐性の，殺菌性の	intracellular	細胞内の
aqueous	水成の	invalid	無効な
asymptomatic	無症候性の	leafless	葉のない
benign	良性の	malaria	マラリア
contradiction	否定，矛盾	malignant	悪性の
contrary	反対の	malnutrition	栄養失調
counterstain	対比染色する	modify	修飾する
counterview	反論	motionless	静止した
deforestation	森林伐採	negate	否定する
degassed	ガスが抜かれた	negligible	無視してよい
dehydrate	脱水する	neolithic	新石器時代の
deionized	脱イオンの	nonabrasive	摩擦をひき起こさない
detox	体内浄化する	nonfat	無脂
dislocation	脱臼	paleolithic	旧石器時代の
dysfunction	機能障害	previously	以前に
dyspepsia	消化不良	pseudonym	筆名
dystrophy	発育異常, 萎縮症, 栄養失調	pseudopodia	仮足，擬足
enable	可能にする，許可する	pseudoscience	擬似科学
encode	暗号に書き直す	purify	精製する
endocrine	内分泌の	quantify	量を計る，定量化する
enlarge	拡張する	quasi drugs	医薬部外品
eubacteria	真正細菌	quasicrystal	準結晶
eupepsia	消化良好	respectively	それぞれの
euphemism	婉曲語法	sonicated	超音波処理した
exchange	交換する	subsequently	その後
exocrine	外分泌の	troublesome	煩わしい
false-positive	偽陽性の	unaltered	不変の
flawless	完璧な	unanalyzable	分析できない
heterogenous	異種起源の，(cf. heterogeneous)不均一の	undo	元に戻す
		unsuccessful	失敗した
homogenous	同種の，(cf. homogeneous)均一の	useful	有用な

(speaker icon) Track 24

Unit
3

Unit 4   1. Reading

Class _____   I.D. _____   Name _____   check

A. Read the text and mark T if the statement is true. Mark F if the statement is false and rewrite the sentence.

1. (T   F)   Blood coagulation is always caused by vascular injury.

_____

2. (T   F)   The four major events introduced in Paragraph 1 describe hyperlipidemia.

_____

3. (T   F)   Hemostasis starts with the gathering of platelets at the site of a damaged blood vessel.

_____

4. (T   F)   Collagen flows in the blood with platelets and other blood cells.

_____

5. (T   F) TXA_2 released by platelets is categorized as an eicosanoid.

_____

6. (T   F)   "Cascade" in this text means a small waterfall.

_____

7. (T   F)   Fibrin clot formation in response to tissue injury is the result of the intrinsic pathway.

_____

8. (T   F)   VLDLs and chylomicrons are lipoprotein particles.

_____

9. (T   F)   Hyperlipidemia can be a cause of atherosclerosis.

_____

Unit

4

B. Listen to the recording and write the answers below.

1.

2.

3.

C. Answer the following questions using the information in the reading.

1. What happens in the initial phase of hemostasis ?

2. What is the role of thrombin in the second phase ?

3. Explain white thrombus and red thrombus.

4. What happens to the clot in the final event ?

Unit 4　2. **Language focus**

Class _____　I.D. _____　Name _____

A. Read the sentences below and indicate the purpose, sequence phrase and procedure, using the notation system in the box below.

> 1. purpose： _____
> 2. sequence phrase： (　　　　)
> 3. procedure 1： 1_____
>   procedure 2： 2_____
>   ⋮

1. To test pluripotency *in vivo*, we transplanted human iPS cells (clone 201B7) subcutaneously into dorsal flanks of immunodeficient (SCID) mice.

   (Takahashi *et al.*, 2007： 866)

   Unit
   4

2. Mononuclear cells were isolated from whole blood.

3. In order to make invisible ink, we prepared a piece of white construction paper, a cotton swab, a lemon, a bowl, and a hand-held hair dryer. Prior to the procedure, the lemon was cut in half and the juice was squeezed out. To begin with, we put the lemon juice in a bowl. Next, we dipped the cotton swab into the juice and then wrote a message on the paper. The juice disappeared as we wrote. Once we've finished writing our message, we turned on the hair dryer (low speed) and blew the hot air onto the paper. As the lemon juice dried, it turned brown. As a result, the invisible message was visible again.

B. Paraphrase sentences 1 and 2 above using your own words. For 3, choose two sentences and rewrite them. (1～4)

1. Paraphrase： _____

   _____

2. Paraphrase： _____

   _____

3. Sentence 1: _____

   Paraphrase: _____

   _____

4. Sentence 2: _____

   Paraphrase: _____

   _____

C. Fill in the blanks. Listen to the recording and check your answers.

1. (_____), scientists studied 5 men and 5 women.
   Hint: The underlined part shows the purpose of the research.

2. (_____), the catheters are removed, and the patients can
   go home.
   Hint: The underlined part shows a stage of the procedure.

3. (_____), electrical tests are conducted on the heart.
   Hint: The electrical tests —→ The procedure

4. Artificial trans fats are formed (_____) liquid oils are turned into solid fats.
   Hint: Liquid oils are turned into solid fats —→ Artificial trans fats are formed

5. (_____), the scientists used a new and sophisticated technique.
   Hint: The underlined part shows the purpose of the research.

D. Dictation: Listen to the recording and write what you hear.

1. _____

2. _____

Unit 4 3. Vocabulary

check

Class _____ I.D. _____ Name _____

A. Choose appropriate words/phrases from the box below to complete the sentences.

1. Blood (   ) is a complex process that involves a (   ) of events that occur in a set order.

2. When you get an injury, platelets are (   ) by thrombin and (   ) at the injury site.

3. In order to control blood loss from a cut on the skin, the (   ) of blood (   ) occurs so blood flow lessens.

4. Human blood is (   ) of plasma, (   ), red blood cells, and white blood cells.

5. One type of stroke is caused by bleeding in the brain (   ) to the (   ) of a blood vessel.

Unit
4

activated	aggregate	cascade	coagulation
comprised	constriction	platelets	rupture
subsequent	vessels		

B. Match the beginnings (1 to 5) to the endings (a to e) to complete the following sentences.

1. Hemostasis refers to (　)

2. Activated platelets (　)

3. When the tissue is repaired, (　)

4. Anti-coagulants enable (　)

5. Maintaining good vascular health through regular exercise is (　)

a. normal blood flow is resumed.

b. the formation of a thrombus or blood clot.

c. the dissolution of blood clots.

d. induce the secretion of many kinds of proteins.

e. paramount for long life.

C. Underline the affixes in the following words, and then write the meaning of the affixes and the words.

1. agent　　affix: [　　　　] 　meaning: [　　　　　　　　　　]

2. fluid　　affix: [　　　　] 　meaning: [　　　　　　　　　　]

3. alkane　　affix: [　　　　] 　meaning: [　　　　　　　　　　]

4. solution　　affix: [　　　　] 　meaning: [　　　　　　　　　　]

5. ethylene　　affix: [　　　　] 　meaning: [　　　　　　　　　　]

D. Dictation: Listen to the recording and write the words or sentences you hear.

1. _____

2. _____

3. _____

4. _____

5. _____

Unit 4 | 4. Reading glossary

🔊 Track 25

abnormal	異常な，異常性の
accommodate	適応させる，順応させる，収容する
activate	活性化する，賦活化する，賦活する
activated platelet	活性化血小板
additional	付加的な，追加の，さらなる
ADP	アデノシン二リン酸
aggregate	凝集する
atherosclerosis	アテローム性動脈硬化
bind	結合する
blood clotting	血液凝固，凝血
blood flow	血流，血流量，血液流量
cascade	カスケード（一連の増幅的な段階反応）
chylomicron	カイロミクロン（食事性脂質を輸送する血漿リポタンパク質）
clinically	臨床的に
clot	血餅，血塊，凝血塊，凝血する，凝固する
clotting factor	凝固因子
clump	集まる，凝集する
coagulation	凝固，凝析，凝血，血液凝固，凝血塊
collagen	コラーゲン，膠原質（骨や軟骨などに多い細胞外繊維状タンパク質）
complex	複雑な，複合体，錯体
comprise	（部分が全体を）構成する，（全体が部分を）含む
constriction	狭窄，収縮，収斂
contact	接触
contain	含む，含有する
continued	継続した
converge	収束する
demonstrate	実証する，立証する，証明する，示す
dissolution	溶解，融解，（構成成分への）分解
dissolve	溶解する，溶ける，溶かす
distinct	特徴的な，（明確に）異なる，明瞭な，明確な
eicosanoid	エイコサノイド（生理活性を有する炭素数 20 の不飽和脂肪酸関連物質の総称）
endothelial	内皮の
entrap	捕捉する，封入する
expose	曝露する，露出する，露光する，被曝する，曝す

Unit

4

extrinsic	外因性の，外的な
fibrin	線維素，フィブリン（血液凝固系の生成物）
fibrin clot	フィブリン血栓，フィブリン塊
fibrinogen	線維素原，フィブリノーゲン（血液凝固第Ⅰ因子）
flow	流れ
formation	形成
generation	生成，産生，発生，世代
hemostasis	止血
hyperlipidemia	（病名）高脂血症
in response to	～に反応して
in the absence of	非存在下で（c.f., in the presence of）
induce	誘導する，誘発する，誘起する，ひき起こす，導入する
initial	初期の，最初の，初回の，初発性の
initiate	始める
injure	損傷する，傷つける
injury	外傷，損傷
insure	保証する
integrity	完全性（無傷の状態），整合性，統合性
intrinsic	内因性の，内在性の
involve	関与する，関わる
lining	内膜
lipoprotein	リポタンパク質（血漿中に存在する）
loose	ゆるい（比較級 looser- 最上級 loosest）
mesh	網状組織，メッシュ
nucleotide	ヌクレオチド（核酸塩基 ＋ 糖 ＋ リン酸）
numerous	多数の
occur	起こる，発生する，生じる
paramount	最高の
particle	粒子
pathway	経路，パスウェイ
phase	段階，相，期，時期
phospholipid	リン脂質
physiological condition	生理的状態
plasmin	プラスミン（酵素）
platelet	血小板
plug	栓，栓子，プラグ，塞ぐ
primarily	おもに
protein	タンパク質
red blood cell	赤血球
release	放出する，遊離する
relevant	適切な，関連性のある

repair	修復，修復する，直す
resume	再開する，回復する
rupture	破裂，断裂，破裂する
secretion	分泌
serotonin	セロトニン（神経伝達物質；オータコイド）
significance	重要性，意義，有意性
site	部位，サイト
stability	安定性，安定度
stimulating	stimulating〜　〜を促すこと
subsequent	ひき続く，後の
survival	生存
temporary	一時的な，一時の
term	名付ける，用語，期間
thrombin	トロンビン
thrombus	血栓
tissue	（生体の）組織
TXA$_2$	トロンボキサン A$_2$
vascular	血管性の，血管の，脈管の，（植物）維管束の
vessel	血管
vessel wall	血管壁
VLDL	超低密度リポタンパク質（very low density lipoprotein）

Unit
4

Unit 4　5. Word-formation samples

acetic	酢酸の	fluid	流動性の
acidity	酸性度	flux	流動
acrylic	アクリルの	fraction	断片
activity	活性，活性度	glycemia	糖血症
acute	鋭い，急性の	glycerol	グリセロール
adhesion	付着，粘着	glycogen	グリコーゲン
agent	作用物質	hydrate	水和物
alias	別名	hydrophilic	親水性の
alkane	アルカン	hydrophobic	疎水性の
alkene	アルケン	immiscible	混ざらない
alkyne	アルキン	isotope	同位体
alloy	合金	lysemia	溶血
alter	変更する	metamorphosis	変形
boson	ボース粒子，ボゾン	methane	メタン
bromide	臭化物	mixture	混合物
bromite	亜臭素酸塩	mobile	可動性の，流動性のある
carbonic	炭素の，炭酸	morphology	形態学
catalysis	触媒作用	nitrate	硝酸塩
catalyst	触媒	nitrous	窒素の
catalyze	触媒作用を及ぼす	octyne	オクチン
cauldron	大釜	oxidative	酸化的な
cauterize	焼灼する	polyene	ポリエン
cohere	しっかりと結合する	prefix	接頭辞
cohesion	結束，凝集	product	生成物，産物
condense	濃縮する	proton	陽子，プロトン
conduct	行為	reagent	試薬
crystal	水晶，結晶	refract	屈折させる
crystalline	結晶の	saccharide	糖類・サッカライド
deduce	推測する	saturated fatty acid	飽和脂肪酸
density	濃度・密度	saturation binding	飽和結合
ductile	延性のある，柔軟な	solution	溶液
electron	電子	solvent	溶剤，溶媒
element	要素，成分，元素	special	専門の
equilibrium	平衡	spectator	観客
equivalent	同等の，等価	spectrum	スペクトル
ethane	エタン	sulfurous acid	亜硫酸
ethylene	エチレン	sulfuric acid	硫酸
ferric	鉄の，第二鉄の	vacant	空いている
ferrous	第一鉄の	vacuous	中身が空の，真空の
fission	分裂	vacuum	真空
fixture	備品	volatile	揮発性の
fluctuate	変動する	water-soluble	水溶性の

Unit
4

Unit 5   1. Reading

Class _____   I.D. _____   Name _____

A. Read the text and mark T if the statement is true. Mark F if the statement is false and rewrite the sentence.

1. (T   F)   Acesulfame–K (ACE) is a volatile and irritating inorganic substance often found in swimming pools.

_____

2. (T   F)   The authors of this research paper conducted a study to find out how much ACE is contained in hot tubs and swimming pools.

_____

3. (T   F)   The reason why ACE was chosen was because ACE is a highly reactive compound.

_____

4. (T   F)   The researchers assume the amount of ACE corresponds to the amount of urine in pools and hot tubs.

_____

5. (T   F)   The samples of this study were taken from cities in the US.

_____

6. (T   F)   No ACE was found in tap water samples.

_____

7. (T   F)   The researchers compared the amount of ACE in the samples from the swimming pools, hot tubs and tap water.

_____

8. (T   F)   The water samples were collected over 10 years.

_____

9. (T   F)   ACE is often used in food and drinks instead of sugar.

_____

Unit

5

B. Listen to the recording and write the answers below.

1.

2.

3.

C. Briefly describe the measurements taken and the instruments used in the chart below.

Measurement (Unit)	Instrument
Temperature (°C, K, °F)	Thermometer

Unit 5   2. Language focus

check

Class _____   I.D. _____   Name _____

A. Read the sentences below and indicate each part of the description of the method, using the notation system in the box below.

> 1. materials / instrument: [   ]
> 2. a performing verb: _____
> 3. condition: (   )
> 4. purpose: to/for _____

1. A scanning electron microscope was used to magnify a single hair cell from the mouse ear.

2. These muscle-specific FLCN knockout mice were crossbred with other knockout mice that lacked the PPARGC1A gene.

3. To identify the unknown organism, the tissue sample was incubated and tested for bacteria and viruses.

4. To measure insect diversity in coffee fields, insects were collected for several months.

Unit
5

B. Paraphrase each sentence above using one of the sentence patterns introduced in this unit. (1 ~ 4)

1. _____

_____

2. _____

_____

3. _____

_____

4. _____

_____

C. Fill in the blanks. Listen to the recording and check your answers.

1. A vane anemometer (   ) (   ) (   ) to record temperature and airflow speed minute-by-minute. [set up]

2. A centrifuge (   ) (   ) to separate the mixed substances by spinning them. [use]

3. Cooked sushi rice (   ) (   ) (   ) a syrup of salt, vinegar, and sugar that had been heated. [mix]

4. Cesium (   ) (   ) (   ) a solid material with a process that used a chemical reaction. [turn into]

D. Dictation: Listen to the recording and write what you hear.

1. _____

2. _____

Unit 5 3. Vocabulary

Class _____ I.D. _____ Name _____

check

A. Choose appropriate words/phrases from the box below to complete the sentences.

1. (   ) in swimming pools can be (   ) by checking the (   ) of ACE.

2. In order to avoid contamination, you have to use (   ) equipment.

3. Chemical markers are used to (   ) harmful substances, such as asbestos, before they enter our (   ).

4. Some bacteria break down (   ) waste products to release energy. This (   ) causes nitrogen to be released.

concentration	decomposition	detect	detected
nitrogenous	sterile	tap water	urine excretion

B. Underline the verbs in the following text. Then complete the sentences by choosing the most appropriate item from the box below.

at by in（3カ所） into（3カ所） on

Basic PCR Protocol（Excerpt from Lorenz, 2012）（1〜6）

1. Place a 96 well plate (   ) the ice bucket as a holder for the 0.2 ml thin walled PCR tubes.

2. Pipette the following PCR reagents in the following order (   ) a 0.2 ml thin walled PCR tube: Sterile water, 10X PCR buffer, dNTPs, $MgCl_2$, primers, and template DNA.

3. (   ) a separate 0.2 ml thin walled PCR tubes add all the reagents.

4. Taq DNA polymerase is typically stored (   ) a 50% glycerol solution and for complete dispersal (   ) the reaction mix requires gentle mixing of the PCR reagents (   ) pipetting up and down at least 20 times.

5. Put caps (   ) the 0.2 ml thin walled PCR tubes and place them (   ) the
   thermal cycler. Once the lid to the thermal cycler is firmly closed start the program.

6. When the program has finished, the 0.2 ml thin walled PCR tubes may be removed and
   stored (   ) 4 °C.

C. Underline the affixes in the following words, and then write the meaning of the
   affixes and the words.

1. ambulance   affix: [   ]   meaning: [   ]

2. dorsiflex   affix: [   ]   meaning: [   ]

3. operation   affix: [   ]   meaning: [   ]

4. transect   affix: [   ]   meaning: [   ]

5. contagious   affix: [   ]   meaning: [   ]

6. erythrocyte   affix: [   ]   meaning: [   ]

7. postmortem   affix: [   ]   meaning: [   ]

8. thyroid   affix: [   ]   meaning: [   ]

D. Dictation: Listen to the recording and write the words or sentences you hear.

1. _____

2. _____

3. _____

4. _____

5. _____

Unit 5　4. Reading glossary

◀)) Track 27

ACE	（食品添加物）アセスルファム K（acesulfame-K）
adverse	有害な，反対の，反する
amine	（化合物）アミン
application	適用，応用
assessment	アセスメント，影響評価，評価，判定
avoid	回避する，避ける
carryover	もち越し汚染，もち越されたもの，キャリーオーバー
chlorine	塩素
collect	採取する，集める
complete	完全な，徹底的な
concentration	濃度，濃縮
consumption	摂取
contamination	混入，汚染，コンタミネーション，（俗）コンタミ
contribution	関与
control	調節，制御，対照（実験）
DBP	消毒副生成物（disinfectant byproduct）
decomposition	分解，腐敗
desirable	望ましい
detectable	検出可能な，検出できるほどの
determine	測定する，定量する
develop	開発する
disposable	使い捨ての，ディスポーザブルの
dissolve	溶解する，溶ける，溶かす
edge	端，ふち
effect	影響，作用
epidemiological	疫学的な，疫学上の
estimate	見積もる，推定する
excretion	排泄，排出
exposure	曝露
filter	フィルターをかける，濾過する
-fold	（接尾辞）…倍の
form	形成する，組成する
future	将来，今後
gallon	（単位）ガロン
grab sample	グラブサンプル，試料の収集法
high-throughput	大量処理の，高処理の
hot tub	ホットタブ，温水浴槽
HPLC-MS/MS	高速液体クロマトグラフ（HPLC）と三連四重極型質量分析計（MS/MS）を組合わせた装置（high-performance liquid chromatography with tandem mass spectrometry）
ideal	理想的な，理想，（目的に）ぴったりの

Unit

5

impact	影響，インパクト
inject	注入する
input	注入された，入力，投入
instrument	装置，器具，機器
irritating	刺激性の
level	値，レベル，水準，度合
marker	マーカー，標識
material	材料，資料
method	方法，手法
Millipore	（社名）ミリポア
municipal	地方自治体の，市政機関の
nitrogenous	窒素性の
occurrence	現れること，出現，存在
organic	有機の
over	（期間）わたって
polystyrene	（プラスチック）ポリスチレン
preconcentration	予備濃縮
PVDF	（フィルターの素材）ポリフッ化ビニリデン（polyvinylidene difluoride）
range	（…から…に／…の間に）およぶ，わたる，範囲
react	（with/to）…に反応する
recreational	娯楽の，娯楽的な
report	報告する
resistant	抵抗力がある，耐性がある，抵抗性の，耐性の
sample	試料，検体，標本，サンプル
sequential analysis	逐次解析，系列，分析
source	源，供給源
stable	安定な，安定性のある，安定的な
sterile	無菌の，殺菌した
sweetener	甘味料
synthetic	合成の
tap water	水道水
triplicate	三通りの，三組の
vial	バイアル，小瓶，小ビン
volatile	揮発性の，揮発の
volume	容積，体積，量
widespread	普及している，一般に広がった

Unit 5 5. Word-formation samples

Track 28

ambulatory	歩行の，外来，遊走
abstinent	自制的，禁止
amble	ゆっくり歩く
ambulance	救急車
amoeboid	アメーバ様の
anatomy	解剖学
appendectomy	虫垂切除術
cognitive	認識の
congest	うっ血させる
conifer	針葉樹
conjunctive tissue	結合組織
conscious	気づいて
conservationist	保護主義者
contact	接触，接点
contagious	伝染性の
cryptic	隠れた，潜在性の，陰性
cryptozoa	隠潜動物
deltoid	三角筋
diagnosis	診断
digest	消化する
disjunction	分離，分裂
dissect	解剖する 分析する
dorsiflex	手首，足首を 反らすように曲げる
durable	耐久性のある
dura mater	硬膜
emolliate	柔らかくする
endoscope	内視鏡
erythroblast	赤芽球
erythrocyte	赤血球
esophagus	食道
evident	明らかな
exhale	吐き出す
export	輸出，排出
flexible	しなやかな，柔軟な 変形しやすい
flexor	屈筋
geotropism	屈地性
germicide	殺菌剤
gestation	妊娠，形成
halitosis	口臭，口臭症
herbivorous	草食性の
immigration	移住
immunization	予防接種
immunology	免疫学
import	輸入，取込む
incision	切込み・切開
indigestion	消化不良
infer	推測する，暗示する
innate	生来の
intercept	遮断する
juvenile	若年性の
lumpectomy	乳腺腫瘍摘出手術
macrophage	マクロファージ
microtome	マイクロトーム
migrate	移住する
migratory	移住性の
mollify	和らげる，鎮める
mollusk	軟体動物
mortal	致命的な，死すべき
mutagen	突然変異原
mutant	突然変異体
natal	出生の
native	出生地の
neonate	新生児
neoplasm	新生物（腫瘍）
olfaction	嗅覚
olfactory	嗅覚の
operation	作用，働き，手術，操作
orthopedic	整形外科的な
orthoptera	直翅類，バッタ類
pesticide	殺虫剤
phagocyte	食細胞
portable	移動用の，持ち運び可能な
postnatal	出生後の

prescription	処方箋	sensor	検出器
preserve	維持する	sensory	感覚の
prognosis	予後	sessile	固着の
receptor	受容体	steroid	ステロイド
refer	指す，参照する	stethoscope	聴診器
rejuvenate	若返らせる	tactile	触覚の
residue	残留物，残渣，残基	tendon	腱
respiration	呼吸	thyroid	甲状腺
retention	保留，保持	transect	横切する，切除する
reverse transcriptase	逆転写酵素	tropomyosin	トロポミオシン
revise	修正する	vital	生命の，致命的な，活気のある
sedentary	定住性，固着性		
sensation	感覚	vitamin	ビタミン

Unit 6   1. Reading

Class _____   I.D. _____   Name _____

A. Read the text and mark T if the statement is true. Mark F if the statement is false and rewrite the sentence.

1. (T   F)   The researchers collected samples from swimming pools and hot tubs at 8 facilities including private facilities in city 1.

_____

2. (T   F)   The concentration of ACE in the pool sample was the highest in SP 8 in city 2.

_____

3. (T   F)   Hot tub samples from the two cities can be divided into two groups according to the level of ACE concentration: one from 70 to 100 ng/L and the other from 2220 to 7110 ng/L.

_____

4. (T   F)   The factors that influence the concentration level of ACE include the water temperature.

_____

5. (T   F)   Although more attention is supposed to be paid to the hygiene of hot tubs, some hot tubs in this study contained a significant amount of ACE.

_____

6. (T   F)   The ACE concentration level in HT5 was 571 times greater than that in HT8.

_____

7. (T   F)   The researchers were not surprised at the findings about the ACE concentration levels of the two cities' tap water.

_____

8. (T   F)   The water for the two cities' tap water comes from the same source.

_____

9. (T   F)   The average ACE concentration in tap water collected in city 1 was higher than that in city 2.

_____

10. (T   F)   The ACE concentration of the tap water samples in the two cities is similar to that of some Albertan well water samples.

_____

Unit

6

B. Listen to the recording and write the answers below.

1.

2.

3.

C. Read the text on pp. 90-92. Complete the notes below.

Figure 2	
Figure 2a Location What were the samples ? Where did they collect them ?	
Figure 2b Location What were the samples ? Where did they collect them ?	
Statistical analysis What did they compare ? The result of the analysis	
The reason for the difference in ACE concentrations of tap water in the two cities.	

Unit 6	2. Language focus		check

Class _____ I.D. _____ Name _____

A. Read the sentences below and indicate each part of the description of the results, using the notation system in the box below.

> 1. measurement / statistical analysis: [   ]
> 2. a verb to indicate the result: _____
> 3. data: (   )
> 4. table / figure: (   )
> 5. results: {   }

1. The wind speeds of Super Typhoon Hagibis were from 161 mph up to 335 mph.

2. The most sensitive range of bat hearing was 15 kHz to 90 kHz (kilohertz).

3. To check the normal distribution of the data, skewness and kurtosis were analyzed, both of which were within ± 2 for all 6 variables.

4. The combined average of ACE concentration in each city's tap water was found to be statistically different using an unpaired Student's t-test: ($p < 0.001$).

B. Paraphrase each sentence above using one of the sentence patterns introduced in this unit. (1 ~ 4)

Unit 6

1. _____

   _____

2. _____

   _____

3. _____

_____

4. _____

_____

C. Categorize the following verbs according to the type of change they describe.

bottom out	decline	decrease	dip	drop
fall	flatten out	fluctuate	flutter	go down
go up	grow	increase	keep pace	
keep the same trend	level off	occupy (ratio)	plateau	plunge
reach a low	reach a peak	reduce	remain constant	remain flat
remain still	rise	stabilize	stagnate	stay flat
turn upward	undulate	zig-zag		

up	down	up and down	level

Unit 6   3. Vocabulary

Class _____   I.D. _____   Name _____

A. Choose appropriate words/phrases from the box below to complete the sentences.

1. The figure shows the (   ) level of ACE contained in the water in swimming pools in the whole area.

2. The difference between the two samples was (   ) significant.

3. If your intake of ACE increases, you will see a (   ) increase in the level of ACE in your urine.

4. I like natural sweeteners including honey and maple syrup, (   ) my sister prefers synthetic sweeteners such as ACE and aspartame (APM).

5. Every person's DNA is (   ).

6. Use a (   ) ratio of 1 part water to 1 part vinegar to clean your kitchen.

7. The table shows a greater (   ) in ACE concentrations in hot tubs than pools.

8. The study determined that typically hot tub water in public (   ) is (   ) more often than pool water.

average	corresponding	dilution	facilities	replaced
statistically	unique	variation	whereas	

Unit

6

B. Graph reading exercises

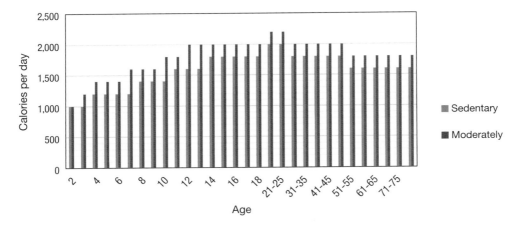

Figure. (Title) _____

1. What kind of graph is this ?

_____

2. Choose an appropriate title for the graph and write it under the graph.

   a. Daily calorie needs by age for sedentary and moderately active females

   b. Sedentary and moderate needs of daily calories by active females' of various ages

   c. Females' daily needs of sedentary and moderately active calories by age

   d. Sedentary and moderately active females' by age of needs of daily calorie

3. Which part of the graph is the x-axis ?

4. Which part of the graph is the y-axis ?

5. Where is the legend ? Circle it. What is it called in Japanese ?

C. Dictation: Listen to the recording and write the words or sentences you hear.

1. _____

2. _____

Unit 6 — 4. Reading glossary

Track 29

analyze	分析する，解析する
associated with	～関連している
collect	収集する，採取する，集める，捕集する
combined	合わせた，結合した
comparable	匹敵する，同等の，比較できる
concentration	濃度，濃縮
contain	含む，含有する，包む
corresponding	対応している，一致している
cycling	サイクル，回路，周期（本文では水の入れ換え周期）
detect	検出する，検知する
determine	決定する，特定する，確定する，判定する，測定する，定量する
dilution	希釈，希釈度，希釈法
discussion	考察，討論
facility	施設，設備
fresh water	淡水
indicate	指し示す，示す，意味する，指摘する，指示する
issue	問題
location	場所
maintain	維持する，継続する
management	管理
prevent	防ぐ，防止する，阻止する，妨げる
replace	置換する，交換する
represent	…を表す，述べる，説明する，表現する，代表する，となる
residence	住居，居住地
sampling	サンプリング，検体採取，試料採取，（統計）標本抽出
snapshot	snapshot in time ある一瞬のこと
t-test	t 検定（Student's t-検定）
table	表，テーブル
typically	典型的に
unique	独特の，特有の，唯一の
variation	変動，多様性，差異

Unit
6

Unit 6 5. Word-formation samples

biology	生物学	dystrophy	ジストロフィー, 栄養失調症
chromosome	染色体		
leukocyte	白血球	insecticide	殺虫剤
aquarium	水族館, 水槽	monogamy	一夫一婦主義
herbivore	草食動物	gamete	配偶子
oocyte	卵母細胞	cytogenic	細胞発生の
antitoxin	抗毒素	genotype	遺伝子型
protozoa	原生生物	genealogy	家系・血筋
pediatrician	小児科医	genetics	遺伝学
android	人造人間	appendicitis	虫垂炎
hominid	ヒト科動物の	arthritis	関節炎
cephalic	頭部の	lyse	溶解する
ectoderm	外胚葉	hemolysis	溶血
bipedal	二足歩行の	hydrolysis	加水分解
somatic cell	体細胞	methodology	方法論
lysosome	リソソーム	epidemiology	疫学
neuron	神経細胞	photosynthesis	光合成

◀)) Track 30

Unit

6

Words and phrases frequently used to describe data

1. Types of analysis　（データ分析の方法）

   ①　qualitative analysis　（定性分析）　　②　quantitative analysis　（定量分析）

2. Description of data（descriptive statistics）　（記述統計）

   ①　average　（平均，一般的には mean を指す）　⑥　distribution　（分布）

   ②　mean　（平均値＝算術平均値）　⑦　standard deviation　（標準偏差）

   ③　median　（中央値）　⑧　standard error　（標準誤差）

   ④　mode　（最頻値）　⑨　skewness　（歪度）

   ⑤　variance　（分散）　⑩　kurtosis　（尖度）

3. Data analyses　（統計）

   ①　parametric measure　（パラメトリック検定，母集団の分布による検定）　④　ANOVA　（Analysis of variance）（分散分析）

   ⑤　correlation　（相関）

   ②　nonparametric measure　（ノンパラメトリック，分布によらない検定）　⑥　regression analysis　（回帰分析）

   ⑦　factor analysis　（因子分析）

   ③　t-test　（Student's t-test）（t 検定）　⑧　chi-squared test　（χ^2 test, カイ二乗検定）

4. Graphs　（グラフ）

   ①　bar graph　（棒グラフ）　③　pie chart　（円グラフ）

   ②　line graph　（線グラフ）　④　scatter plot　（散布図）

5. Terms used in statistics　（統計用語）

   ①　independent variable　（独立変数）　⑤　P-value, p-value　（P 値＝有意確率）

   ②　dependent variable　（従属変数）　⑥　null hypothesis　（H_0）（帰無仮説）

   ③　N, n　（母集団のサイズ N，標本数 n）　⑦　alternative hypothesis　（H_1）（対立仮説）

   ④　F-value　（F 値＝統計量）

Unit

6

Workbook
References

Abozenadah, H., Bishop, A., Bittner, S., Lopez, O., Wiley, C., and Flatt, P.M. (2017). Consumer Chemistry: How Organic Chemistry Impacts our Lives. Chapter 8: Alkenes, Alkynes and Aromatic Compounds, https://wou.edu/chemistry/courses/online-chemistry-textbooks/ch105-consumer-chemistry/ch105-chapter-108/.

Buszczak, M., Signer, R.A., and Morrison, S.J. (2014). Cellular differences in protein synthesis regulate tissue homeostasis. Cell *159*, 242–251.

Ghaedi, M., Niklason, L.E., and Williams, J. (2015). Development of Lung Epithelium from Induced Pluripotent Stem Cells. Curr Transplant. Rep. *2*, 81–89.

Hagen, J., Zimmerman, R., Goetz, C., Bonnevier, J., Houchins, J.P., Reagan, K., and Kalyuzhny, A.E. (2015). Comparative Multi-Donor Study of IFNgamma Secretion and Expression by Human PBMCs Using ELISPOT Side-by-Side with ELISA and Flow Cytometry Assays. Cells *4*, 84–95.

Lawton, M.P., and Nahemow, L. (1973). Ecology and the aging process. In The psychology of adult development and aging, pp. 619–674.

Li, X., Dunn, J., Salins, D., Zhou, G., Zhou, W., Schussler-Fiorenza Rose, S.M., Perelman, D., Colbert, E., Runge, R., Rego, S., *et al.* (2017). Digital Health: Tracking Physiomes and Activity Using Wearable Biosensors Reveals Useful Health–Related Information. PLoS Biol. *15*, e2001402.

Lorenz, T.C. (2012). Polymerase chain reaction: basic protocol plus troubleshooting and optimization strategies. J. Vis. Exp. e3998.

Pironi, L., Arends, J., Baxter, J., Bozzetti, F., Pelaez, R.B., Cuerda, C., Forbes, A., Gabe, S., Gillanders, L., Holst, M., *et al.* (2015). ESPEN endorsed recommendations. Definition and classification of intestinal failure in adults. Clin. Nutr. *34*, 171–180.

Ruderman, N.B., and Saha, A.K. (2006). Metabolic syndrome: adenosine monophosphate-activated protein kinase and malonyl coenzyme A. Obesity (Silver Spring) *14 Suppl 1*, 25S–33S.

Ruotsalainen, V., Ljungberg, P., Wartiovaara, J., Lenkkeri, U., Kestila, M., Jalanko, H., Holmberg, C., and Tryggvason, K. (1999). Nephrin is specifically located at the slit diaphragm of glomerular podocytes. Proc. Natl. Acad. Sci. U S A *96*, 7962–7967.

Takahashi, K., Tanabe, K., Ohnuki, M., Narita, M., Ichisaka, T., Tomoda, K., and Yamanaka, S. (2007). Induction of pluripotent stem cells from adult human fibroblasts by defined factors. Cell *131*, 861–872.

Takahashi, K., and Yamanaka, S. (2006). Induction of pluripotent stem cells from mouse embryonic and adult fibroblast cultures by defined factors. Cell *126*, 663–676.

Warnhoff, K., Roh, H.C., Kocsisova, Z., Tan, C.H., Morrison, A., Croswell, D., Schneider, D.L., and Kornfeld, K. (2017). The Nuclear Receptor HIZR-1 Uses Zinc as a Ligand to Mediate Homeostasis in Response to High Zinc. PLoS Biol. *15*, e2000094.

第 1 版 第 1 刷 2021 年 3 月 10 日 発行
第 2 刷 2023 年 8 月 1 日 発行

ライフサイエンスのための英語
I. 基本スキル編

© 2 0 2 1

編 著 者　　　萩　原　明　子
　　　　　　　小　林　　　薫

発 行 者　　　石　田　勝　彦

発　　行　　株式会社 東京化学同人

東京都文京区千石 3 丁目 36-7（〒112-0011）
電話 03-3946-5311・FAX 03-3946-5317
URL: https://www.tkd-pbl.com/

印 刷　中央印刷株式会社
製 本　株式会社 松岳社

ISBN978-4-8079-0979-7
Printed in Japan

ライフサイエンスのための
英　語
II. プレゼンテーション編

萩原明子・内藤麻緒・小 林　薫 編著
B5 判　184 ページ　定価 2860 円（本体 2600 円＋税）

自然科学系大学生を対象とした半期（12回）の講義を想定した教科書．簡単な例を用いることによって自然科学をテーマにしたプレゼンテーションの基本（スライドの作り方や話し方など）が学べる．スピーキング練習のための動画付．

主要目次 プレゼンテーションとは／プレゼンターとスタディの紹介／背景と研究目的の紹介／使用した材料と研究方法の提示／結果，考察とまとめ／ポスター発表／模範解答／付録（機能表現集／ルーブリック／スクリプトのチェックリスト／プレゼンテーション評価シート／プレゼンテーションメモ）

2023 年 6 月現在（定価は 10 ％税込）